PURE CALISTHENICS
For Beginners

The Essential Guide to Your Fitness Journey

BRUCE

NOLAN

Copyright

Pure Calisthenics for Beginners

Contents

Introduction

Calisthenics are exercises that make use of the body's weight as a form of resistance. And, just like any other form of resistance training, the goal of calisthenics is to promote muscle growth and strength. Originating from the Greek words "kalo", which means *beauty*, and "sthenos," which means *strength*, calisthenics rose into prominence in the 19th century under the father of gymnastics, Freidrich Ludwig Jahn, and fittingly enough, nothing is really a better embodiment of beauty and strength than gymnastics. Since calisthenics uses your body's weight as resistance, it is also known as Bodyweight Exercises. And the big question about bodyweight exercises is how effective they are for building muscle and strength. or if it is as effective as lifting weights. To get a clear understanding of this, we need to know how muscles grow and get stronger.

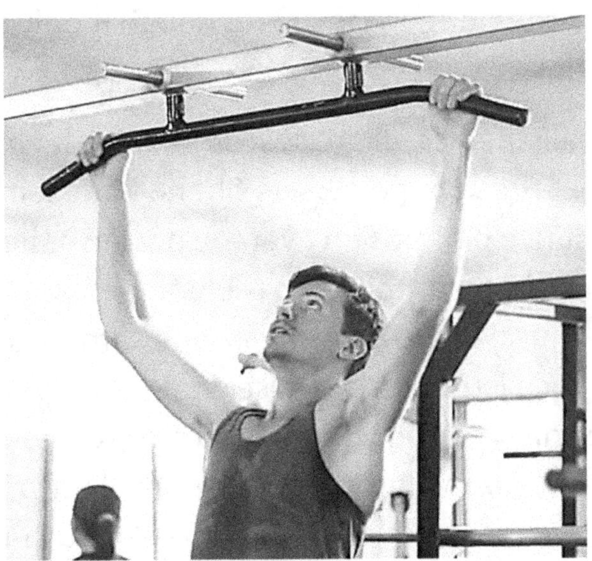

Muscular and strength adaptation occurs when a stimulus or resistance is applied to a corresponding muscle at a high enough intensity to invoke muscular overload. In simpler terms, the more weight you move with your muscles, the more your muscles adapt and become bigger and stronger. However, this doesn't automatically mean that any type of weight movement will work. For instance, although jogging can be very demanding on the heart muscles and promote cardiac muscle growth, it will not promote much skeletal growth, not even in the legs. The issue here is that the stimulus is not strong enough to target all the leg's muscle fibers. The body system has three different muscle fiber types, one of which is used for endurance (Type 1), and the other two are used to provide a great deal of force (Type 2). Since running doesn't require a large amount of force from your legs, Type 2 fibers are hardly fatigued, and not a lot of muscle growth occurs. For this reason, a lot of people don't consider jogging a calisthenic exercise, even though it only utilizes your body's weight.

But other calisthenics exercises do induce a high enough demand to hit those large muscle fibers. For example, people can hardly hit five pull-ups on average because the movement demands all fiber types to fire to the point of exhaustion, thus promoting muscle growth. Push-ups are another good example of a calisthenics exercise that can enhance muscle growth, especially for beginners who struggle to do even 10. But eventually, you will run into the problem of not having enough resistance. As tough as your first 10 push-ups may be, soon they will become an easy warmup. When you start hitting 20, 25, or 30 push-ups easily, then you run into the same problem as described in jogging. Of course, you might then have to modify the push-ups to make them tougher, i.e., by putting your feet on a platform. You are, however, not changing the amount of demand on the muscle groups involved in a standard push-up; instead, you begin shifting the muscles involved in the movement. With elevated push-ups, your anterior shoulders begin to take the brunt of the resistance instead of your chest. You might now be thinking "Why not add some weight to my back?". Well, at this point, it is no longer calisthenics or bodyweight.

The great thing about calisthenics is that it is absolutely free. All you may need is the ground you walk on and areas with solid   structures, i.e., a park with bars. The only time you might have to spend money is on things like suspension systems or gymnastic rings. For beginners, bodyweight exercises will provide all the compound movements that are usually found in a workout program and won't require you to motivate yourself to go to the gym.

Some Misconceptions About Calisthenics

The fitness industry has increasingly acknowledged the numerous advantages of calisthenics, a form of exercise that entails strengthening muscles using one's own body weight. People are beginning to realize that it is entirely feasible to engage in a workout regimen devoid of specialized equipment and still attain results comparable to those achieved through rigorous weightlifting routines.

However, a prevailing misconception persists among many individuals who believe that solely relying on bodyweight exercises is less strenuous and, consequently, less effective than traditional weight-based workouts. To dispel these misconceptions and help fitness enthusiasts recognize the substantial benefits of calisthenics, here are several clarifications:

Calisthenics are for beginners.
Many individuals think that bodyweight exercises are only appropriate for beginners since they should be used as a transition time before moving on to weightlifting, which is the real deal. This idea that lifting weights is more difficult than calisthenics is completely untrue. These two activities each have their own set of advantages and drawbacks. In fact, one should never stop performing bodyweight exercises, regardless of how much success they have in training. These are the motions that are useful in real-life situations. We don't lift as much weight as our bodies do.

Calisthenics won't help you build muscle.
Another prevalent misconception regarding calisthenics is that they are ineffective for muscular building. For this reason, a lot of people try to build up their bodies by lifting weights. This misconception developed because most individuals give up before their bodies are completely exhausted, which is when muscles grow. Mechanical strain and metabolic fatigue

are two factors that lead to muscle gain. The first is taken care of through weightlifting. However, if your goal is to use bodyweight exercises to grow muscles, you should keep going until you are unable to complete another rep with proper form.

If you're not hurting, it's not efficient.
People have a propensity to equate discomfort with progress. They believe their efforts are useless if their muscles feel normal after working out. This 'no pain, no gain' philosophy is, however, completely nonsensical. There is currently no scientific proof that muscles cannot grow when they are not inflamed. The process of burning fat is an invisible one that often results from microtrauma (muscle overuse), which can happen both during bodyweight exercise and when lifting weights.

Calisthenics is meant for the short and slim.
Calisthenics demands that you work your muscles against your own weight. This has led to the notion that these workouts are exclusively beneficial for slim and short people. This is utterly false. While it is true that lighter individuals find it simpler to raise their own bodies during workouts like push-ups, dips, and planks, this does not imply that heavier individuals cannot. In truth, bodyweight exercises can help you slim down and remove stubborn fat. Similar to this, tall people might struggle with pull-ups and planks, but that doesn't mean they shouldn't attempt them.

There should be no days off

Giving yourself a day or two to recover from weight training is crucial because it puts undue strain on your muscles and hammers them into shape. Otherwise, your muscles won't be able to work to their maximum potential. People overlook the value of rests between bodyweight exercises because they view them as a less demanding kind of exercise. This is incorrect because your body's internal mechanisms should be the only factors determining whether or not you take a day off. After a challenging calisthenics workout, take a rest if you don't feel up to it because you won't be able to reap the benefits otherwise.

Calisthenics does not train your legs.
Weightlifting tones your legs more effectively than calisthenics do. This is because the extra weight of dumbbells, kettlebells, or barbells hammers the muscles of the lower body into shape significantly better than conventional squats and lunges. However, this in no way implies that these exercises using only your bodyweight are pointless. They do, albeit to a lesser extent, assist in strengthening the knee joints and expanding the hip range of motion. Additionally, many people find it difficult to perform some versions, such as the pistol squat and box jumps, which call for a higher level of flexibility and fitness.

Calisthenics may be a game changer for your fitness program, and don't trust anyone who tells you differently!

Benefits of Calisthenics

Accessibility: The fact that you can perform the majority of the exercises practically anywhere is one of the best things about calisthenics. Look at what you need to perform push-ups, planks, handstands, sit-ups, and one-legged squats—just the ground. All you need for pull-ups and chin-ups is a bar, and most of the time you will have access to one or a pull-up bar in some form. Effective training can be accomplished without joining a fitness center or lifting weights.

Cost: Engaging in calisthenics is often a cost-effective choice. While you may need to invest in some basic equipment like a pull-up bar, rings, or chalk, the overall expense remains relatively modest. In contrast, a gym membership can be quite pricey, compounded by the fact that it recurs monthly. Opting for calisthenics eliminates the need for a costly gym membership and spares you from purchasing expensive fitness equipment. Consequently, the initial investment in calisthenics is substantially lower.

Develops your Strength: Calisthenics has the remarkable ability to elevate your strength to an entirely new level. It enhances strength, which is not only impressive but also highly practical in daily life. The potential of calisthenics might be underestimated by some, as they are often perceived as inferior to gym-based training in terms of strength development. However, this notion is far from accurate.

Training Multiple Muscle Groups: In calisthenics, there are very few to no movements that will isolate your muscles. The majority of calisthenics routines are essentially compound movements that involve two or more muscular groups at the very least. This can greatly increase the effectiveness of your workouts and improve your overall strength.

Burns Fat: Calisthenics workouts can be beneficial not only for strengthening muscle and strength but also for fat loss. The fact that you will be working out at least a few different categories of muscles also implies that you will burn a lot of calories while performing calisthenics. This particular benefit of calisthenics will undoubtedly appeal to a large number of people.

Improved Flexibility: Whether you like it or not, calisthenics will help you become more flexible. There is simply no getting around this. This is just how bodyweight exercises and calisthenics work.

Improved Posture: Better posture comes with enhanced flexibility. One of the best methods to prevent the negative impacts of an office job is through overall fitness. Rounded shoulders? Hunched back? All of that can be fixed, and it does so through physical exercise. Calisthenics will help you develop your back, abdominal muscles, and erector spinae, which are crucial for good posture.

Versatility: There are calisthenics workouts for all skill levels and talents. Whether you happen to be a complete novice or a seasoned athlete, you will always find an activity that is appropriate for you. Additionally, bodyweight exercises are accessible practically anywhere. There are also numerous variations of bodyweight workouts, so you will never grow bored.

Mental Benefits: Improved sleep, cognitive function, and self-confidence Increases energy, mood, and happiness. Reduces stress.

Joints Friendly: It's no secret that many gym-goers often experience a multitude of injuries, which is one of the major drawbacks of traditional resistance training. These injuries typically result from the use of excessively heavy weightlifting equipment, including machines and barbells. When these tools are misused, they can exert excessive strain on tendons, joints, and other connective tissues. One of the standout advantages of calisthenics lies in its smoother progression, which prevents individuals from attempting exercises that are too demanding before they have acquired sufficient strength. Consequently, calisthenics pose fewer risks to joint health.

It is important to note, however, that while the risk of injury during calisthenics is significantly lower, it is not entirely eliminated. Additionally, calisthenic exercises fall under the category of closed kinetic exercises, indicating that at least one of your body's extremities, such as your hands or feet, remains in constant contact with a stable surface. This feature makes calisthenics highly suitable for physical therapy, as they closely mimic everyday movements. Physiotherapists often recommend calisthenic exercises to enhance joint stability.

Improved Mind-Body Connection: Improvements in the mind-body connection are among physical exercise's highest physical health advantages. There are neurological connections between the brain and the body. These connections serve as a conduit for various messages to move back and forth between the body and the brain. All daily activities carried out by your body are governed by these linkages. Physical exercise can encourage the formation of new synaptic connections and brain plasticity.

Improved Motivation and Mood: There is no doubt that exercise has been linked to higher moods and greater energy. There is, however, a more subdued psychological impact, and that is the simple fact that you will feel confident in yourself. Knowing that you can perform several muscle-ups or pull-ups will do a lot for your self-worth, just like somebody who can bench press 225 pounds will feel wonderful about themselves.

Quick Impact on Abs: Exercises like calisthenics can speed up the process of getting a flat stomach that reveals your sculpted abs. When you work out in the gym, you're more likely to work on your back, arms, and chest. Abs are only used as a supplement to the main exercises. Core training, on the other hand, is included in every single action during a calisthenic workout. Regardless of what bodyweight exercise you do, your abs are always engaged. If you still wish to target your core more effectively, there are numerous calisthenics workouts that will help you tone your abs.

Includes Strength and Cardio training: Calisthenics may provide a great cardio workout alongside strength training.

Perform your routines in a circuit if you want to gain the benefits of strength and cardio exercise from calisthenics. Pick 5–6 calisthenic routines and do them one after the other, with rest periods of 35–45 seconds in between. When you use multiple muscle groups continuously with little rest, your heart rate rises quickly, significantly boosting your cardiovascular endurance.

Can be Done Anywhere and Anytime: Going to the gym is fantastic; going into an atmosphere dedicated to exercise can help you stay motivated. However, there are days when you don't feel like going to the gym or are too busy to stick to your gym plan. Calisthenics allows you to exercise anywhere, at any time, and for no cost. You can do it at home, in the park, or even at work. It removes a variety of obstacles to exercising. Calisthenics require very little gear and very little space. For the majority of the workouts, you already have the equipment—your body—with you.

Drawbacks in Calisthenics

Difficulty Isolating Muscle Groups: In calisthenics, compound motions make up the majority of the workouts. Two or more muscle groups are used in compound motions. For instance, when performing a pull-up, your back, forearms, traps, and biceps will all be involved. You cannot truly isolate a single one from the others. This causes a number of issues if you need to isolate a specific muscle for some reason. You may want to increase the size of your inner biceps, which have an inner and an outer head. Although you can experiment with your chin-ups' breadth grip, you cannot avoid the reality that you will be strengthening your back and other muscles as a result. It is much more challenging to concentrate and isolate the inner biceps.

Calluses: Say good-bye to those lovely and gentle hands. You will develop tough, battle-hardened hands using the rings, pull-up bar, and virtually everything else. You'll wind up with calluses anywhere you never thought it was possible to get them. The bars could be very warm in the summer and very frigid in the winter. Of course, using gloves might be an option, although it is not usually recommended.

The Exercises: The special exercises and movements are the only thing that sets calisthenics apart. However, they do have certain drawbacks. While some exercises, like the push-up, are fairly simple and accessible, others could be exceedingly challenging to perform correctly. Some calisthenics movements might be quite skill-intensive or call for a lot of strength and force. Some exercises, like the planche or even the muscle-up, can be so challenging that it may take a long period of training to master them. This would mean that you would divide these exercises into simpler auxiliary movements in order to perform them. By carrying them out, you'll be able to gradually build up your strength until you reach your goal. The drawback of this is that not everybody will be able to determine which movements and approaches are simpler. Compare this to weightlifting, where you can simply reduce some of the weights to make the activity simpler. There is no way to take off the weight when performing pull-ups.

It is Not Easier than Weightlifting: Many folks might think calisthenics are simpler. Or possibly that no prior knowledge is necessary to perform calisthenics. For instance, not everyone knows how to do push-ups correctly. Push-ups require knowledge and experience, much like a perfect bench press does. Bodyweight workouts can be harmful if done incorrectly, despite the absence of barbells and weights.

Leg Training: The issue with leg training is one of the greatest and most common complaints about calisthenics. In a human body, the muscles in the legs are among the largest. And to train them, you must apply more force or resistance. Your body can only do so much. You might be able to perform 20, 30, or even 50 bodyweight squats even if you have never worked out your legs. High reps can be beneficial, but only to a point. If you want to build muscle, of course, you need enough resistance to allow you to perform fewer squats. The pistol squat is among the best workouts, yet it is still insufficient.

Slower Progress: One notable drawback of calisthenics is its relatively slow rate of progress compared to weightlifting. In the case of weightlifting, you can often witness more rapid advancements in your strength. For example, you might find yourself able to perform dumbbell presses with 50 or even 55 pounds after just two weeks if you were already handling 45 pounds the previous week. This quicker rate of progress is tangible and motivating.

In contrast, calisthenics may require a longer period of time to build the necessary strength before you can truly feel a noticeable difference in your abilities. While progress is still achievable in calisthenics, it may not be as immediately evident as with weightlifting.

CHAPTER ONE
BASICS OF CALISTHENICS

Stretches

Stretching might not be the most thrilling aspect of exercising, but flexibility exercises are crucial to a well-rounded fitness program. Stretching exercises can help you increase your flexibility, relieve tension, and, ultimately, make your workouts—whether they're about strength or aerobic routines—more effective and secure.

During routine daily activity, tight muscles may put an excessive amount of tension on the nearby joints, or they may sustain injury themselves. As we get older, our muscles become shorter and less elastic. Therefore, in order to continue enjoying our abilities painlessly, we need to actively maintain and improve the length of our muscles. Your muscles will become imbalanced if you put a lot of effort into contracting (which shortens) them and never put any effort into stretching (which lengthens) them. Body imbalances raise your risk of injury because they may force some joints and muscles to overcompensate for others that are too tight to engage effectively. This causes discomfort and tension. That's where stretching becomes handy, whether it's about back stretches or leg stretches for upper-body stretches. Stretching and flexibility exercises can help a great deal wherever your muscles are tight.

It's a known fact that stretching is a crucial element of exercise, as it ensures your body is free and ready for the forthcoming action. Also, stretching enhances overall performance and helps you stay injury-free while participating in whatever workout you choose. However, knowing what type of stretching to do is best. Stretches are classified into two types: **Static** and **Dynamic** stretches.

Static Stretches

Static stretches include those whereby you stand, sit, or sleep still for an extended amount of time, up to 45 seconds. Static stretching involves stretching a muscle as far as it may stretch without hurting it, then holding that angle for 20 to 45 seconds. Static stretches should be repeated two to three times. This is an extremely effective method of increasing flexibility. It should be included in your cool-down routine to prevent injury. Static stretching as part of a maintenance stretching routine can also help lower your risk of injury. However, employing static stretching as a warm-up before an athletic competition may have a negative impact on your performance. This is due to the fact that static stretching may impair your body's capacity to react swiftly. In exercises such as vertical jumps, short sprints, balance, and reaction speeds, this condition can persist for up to two hours.

Below are common examples of static stretches:

Posterior capsule stretch: Relax your shoulders, cross one arm over the other, holding it just above the elbow, and slowly draw it toward your body. This stretch targets the rear of the shoulder and will be great for athletes participating in throwing sports like football, baseball, and basketball.

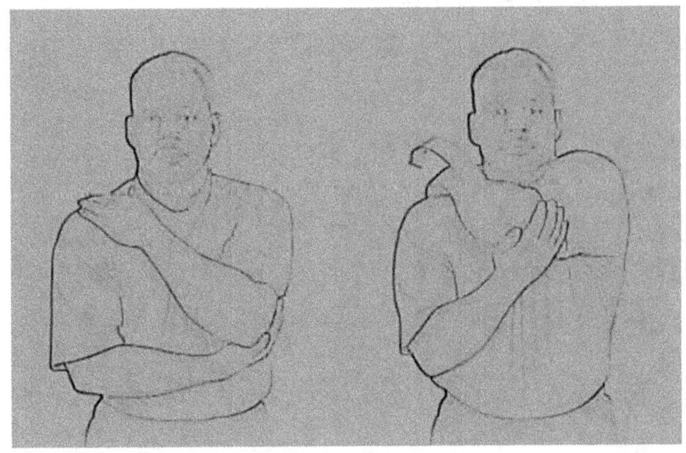

Hamstring stretches: With your hips and feet pointed forward, place one of your legs on a low stool. Lean forward from your hips, keeping a flat back and your knee straight, until you feel a stretch in your thigh. Hamstring stretches help you avoid injuries when running.

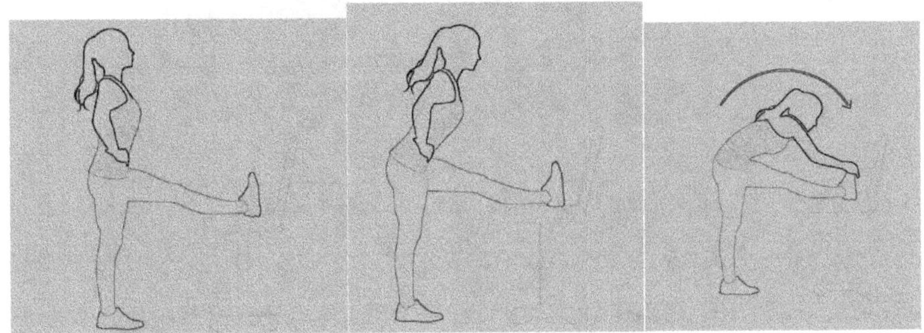

Quadriceps stretch: Grab one ankle from the same side with your hand. To keep your back from hunching, tighten the muscles in your stomach. Bring your ankle up toward your buttocks by extending your thigh rearward, bending your knee, and bringing your ankle up toward your buttocks. Make sure your ankle is parallel to your hip and not tilted outward or inward toward your torso to maintain proper knee-hip alignment. Your front thigh should feel stretched in this position. This stretch is good for the quadriceps muscles.

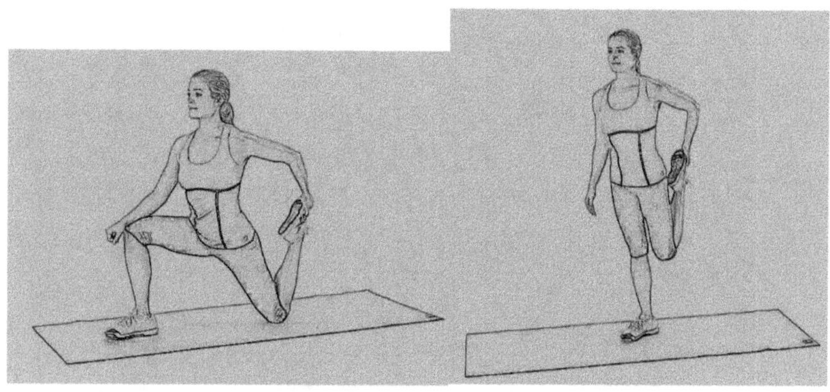

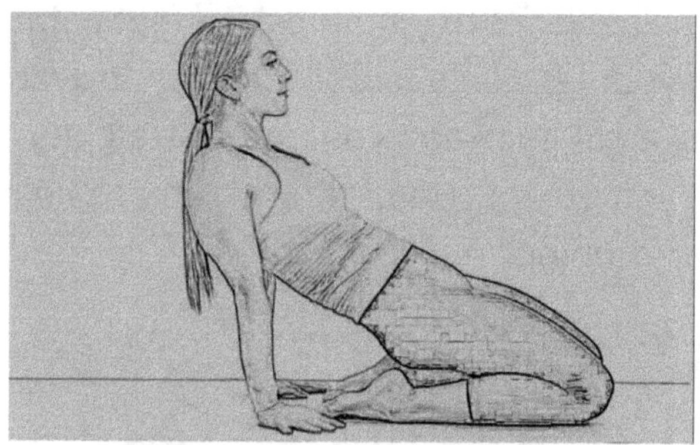

Dynamic Stretches

Dynamic stretches are slow, controlled motions that get your muscles, ligaments, and other soft tissues ready for action and safety. This type of stretching enhances acceleration, speed, and agility. During the stretch, you actively contract your muscles and rotate your joints through their complete range of motion. These practical and athletic movements aid in increasing muscle warmth and reducing stiffness. Dynamic stretches should be adopted as part of your warm-up regimen before any sporting event, competitive or not. A thorough sports warm-up should include 5 to 10 minutes of low- to moderate-intensity swimming, jogging, or cycling, followed by dynamic stretching.

Below are common examples of dynamic stretches:

Torso twist: Stand with your feet forward, as broad as your shoulders, and have your arms by your sides, 90 degrees bent at the elbows. Maintain the same alignment of your feet while slowly rotating your torso from side to side. Don't force the movement, and ensure you're moving through your trunk. This exercise promotes spine mobility and flexibility. Maintaining spine flexibility is specifically important for athletes who participate in throwing and striking sports such as baseball, football, hockey, tennis, and lacrosse.

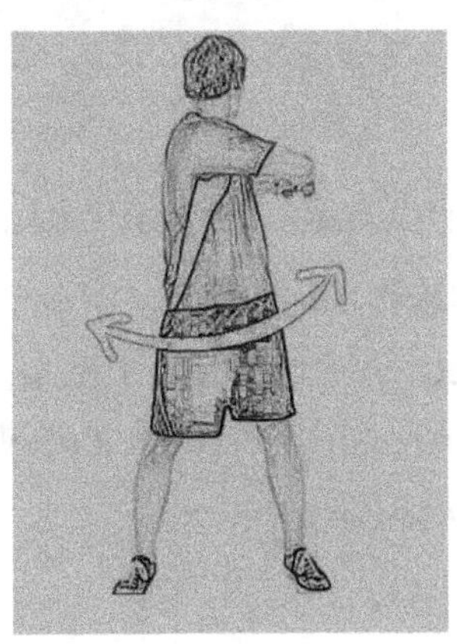

Walking lunge: Standing with your arms akimbo, lunge forward while keeping your front knee parallel to your hip and ankle and lowering your back knee without bringing it into contact with the floor. Avoid letting your front knee cross your front toes. Step forward with the opposing leg, lunging in the same manner as with the rear leg. To prevent your back from arching, keep your abdominal muscles engaged throughout the exercise. All athletes can benefit from doing this, but specifically track and field athletes, soccer players, rugby players, and football players, since it helps to stretch the gluteus, hip flexor muscles, and hamstrings.

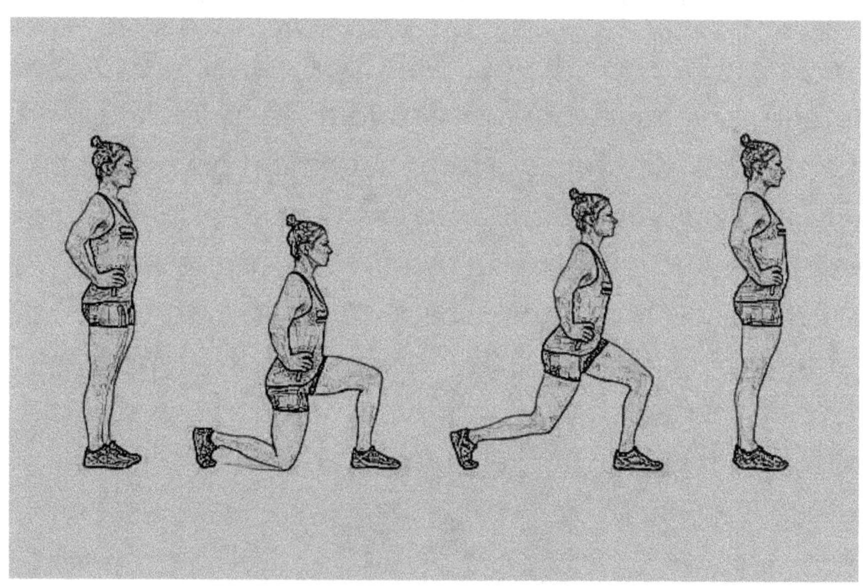

Leg swing: Standing on one leg, mindfully and slowly swing the opposite leg through its entire range of motion in front of and behind you. Keep your abdominal muscles engaged to keep your back from arching. This stretch gets the hip flexors and hamstrings ready for jogging.

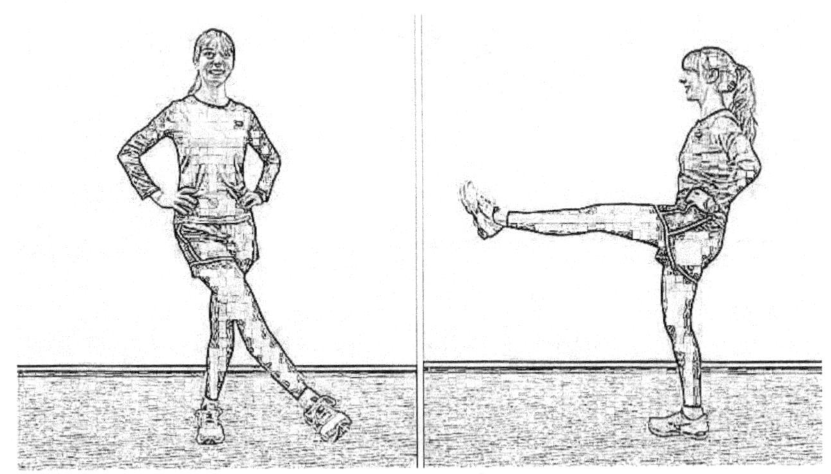

The Concept of Rest

In building muscles, rest doesn't sound particularly exciting, and so it would rarely ever be the cover story of any fitness publication. The message most individuals want to hear is to "do more." After all, that's how you achieve your goals, right? Not really. Your body is worn out and exhausted. Strength development occurs only when you have the chance to recover. And it's not because your brain 'wants' to be stronger that this occurs. No, it doesn't. All it wants to do is adjust to the pressure it must sustain and the stress you subject it to while exercising. Although the human body is an amazing piece of machinery, it has limits. By ignoring rest, you'll quickly reach some of these limits. They are known as injuries.

Important of Rest for Calisthenics

Calisthenics puts a tremendous strain on regions of our bodies that, unless we grew up practicing gymnastics, are not acclimated to such high loads. The ligaments, tendons, and connective tissue that support the wrists, elbows, shoulders, and other joints will get hammered. Additionally, these tissues require significantly more time to heal and recover than muscular tissue. Anyone who is already into calisthenics and trains consistently will be able to describe their elbow ache or the nervy burning they felt in their forearms. The solution is often simple. Focused mobility exercises to loosen up tight tissue and a break from training the motions that initially led to the tissue overload are advised. In other words, take time to rest. These tissues will strengthen and adapt if you do this consistently on a weekly and monthly basis, allowing you to keep working out and getting better. If anything goes wrong, you might be compelled to cease practicing any upper body movements because it will be difficult to avoid putting loads on the injured area, which would impede its healing.

Reasons we often neglect rest
- The fear of losing strength and muscle and gaining weight, hence unending training.
- You want to get better.
- You have a training addiction
- You have a deadline for an upcoming event or competition.

Reasons why we should rest
You will not lose strength in one week; rather, you will develop strength as a result of the adoption process that takes place when you rest. The same holds true for muscular size. Your body mass will be fine if you adjust your diet to meet

your energy needs, i.e., consume less overall energy on non-training days or weeks.

By including organized rest into your program, you will actually progress more since your musculoskeletal and brain systems will heal and adapt to the strain you have been subjecting them to in recent times. This is known as supercompensation. Simply defined, the physiological reaction that makes you stronger than you were before

Addictions to exercise are harmful on a psychological and physical level. You need a break from training to allow your body to heal, gain shape, and maintain mental stability. When preparing for an activity or a sport, you must carefully arrange your training schedule and include adequate rest. If you ignore this, you'll dig yourself a hole that won't help on competition day or in the long run.

As a general rule, you'll need to schedule rest days and de-load weeks.

Rest Days

These are the days of the week when you don't train at all, and such days must be flexible. Can you, for example, get away with only one rest day and six training days each week for four weeks? Or is that level of recuperation insufficient? Consider when your rest days will be and what your 'work:rest' ratio will be. Two days on, one day off. One day on, one day off. It is entirely up to you, your schedule, lifestyle, energy levels, and ability to recuperate. But don't make it a firm decision just yet; it might need to change based on how you feel and how well you've recovered.

It's also important to realize that a regular bodybuilding plan may not be good for a calisthenics beginner due to the extra time required for the ligaments and tendons to recuperate. Longer rest periods between upper-body activities may be necessary to avoid niggles and injury.

De-Load Weeks

If you have been able to complete four or more sessions per week with a reasonable amount of intensity, you should consider the fourth week to be a deloading week. That doesn't imply you should stop training entirely; instead, cut back on a few sessions that week and reduce the volume (total reps) you do. The intensity should stay strong to ensure that you do not lose anything, but a smaller total quantity of work done indicates less stress. You can utilize this extra time to work on other things that will improve your long-term achievement. Mobility, flexibility, and skill practice are all viable possibilities, and the time you spend here will serve as a springboard for the following week.

Cool Down

Finish each workout with a 5-minute cool- down. This could involve stretching activities to calm your muscles and reduce your heart rate. Remember to keep perfect form throughout all of these workouts to avoid injury and maximize results. You can gradually increase the number of reps or sets for each exercise as your fitness level improves. For best results, complete this workout three times each week.

In conclusion, don't consider rest to be an enemy. It's a requirement and necessary for your advancement. Recovery and rest practices will vary from person to person. Your best bet is to plan those rest days and de-loading weeks ahead of time and then stick to them. That requires some self-control. If you can't quite reach that stage, just listen to your body. If your performance in training sessions is stagnant and you're feeling battered, take a deload week and recuperate well enough. This is not laziness or weakness. It is referred to as smart training. It's the same method employed to train great athletes. Their bodies can withstand more weight and stress than others, and most likely more than yours. De-load weeks are a permanent feature in their training schedule, and well, you need them in yours as well if you're training consistently and frequently.

Oscar Wilde once said, "Success is a science; if you create the conditions, you will get the result." One of those conditions in calisthenics is *REST*.

Effective Pre-Workout Rituals

While exercise is promoted as a crucial component of your daily routine, little is mentioned about how to do it properly. Many people focus more on activities than results. They exhaust themselves by attempting difficult actions and their variations while giving little consideration to the results. There is no evidence to suggest that a challenging routine will produce greater results.

In fact, there are occasions when performing easy exercises correctly and with complete focus is significantly more successful than attempting to get the more challenging ones right. Furthermore, you should always work intelligently rather than laboriously. You can take specific actions to improve your overall productivity and results. Include them in your pre-workout regimen and watch your results improve. Here are some pre-workout rituals for result optimization:

Get Enough Rest: Similar to eating well and exercising frequently, getting enough sleep is a crucial component of good health. But nowadays, many people tend to overlook it. Insomnia has become more common in the digital era, which has opened the door for a variety of other diseases to invade the body. This is because sleep strengthens your immune system and enables your muscles to repair the damage they sustained throughout the day. It refills your energy reserves and enables they have to carry out your everyday tasks as efficiently as possible. Get adequate rest before working out to improve your performance.

Timing Pre-Workout Meals: During an exercise, your body requires energy to operate at its peak efficiency. This energy source comes from eating. Feed yourself a nutritious lunch that contains complex carbohydrates or proteins that will help you burn calories rather than store them as negative fat. However, since it will need that much time to be digested, make sure you eat it at least two hours before your workout. On the other hand, it is detrimental to exercise while having a bloated stomach.

Hydrate Yourself: Water aids in the delivery of nutrients and oxygen to all of the cells in the body. It is what causes your muscles to work to their best potential as you exercise. Exercise won't be effective if your body is dehydrated because it won't have the energy to perform demanding activities. Even a two-percent decrease in your body's water level is thought to be able to noticeably affect your health and happiness throughout the day. Having said that, avoid consuming excess water before exercising so that you become immobile. Only consume what your body actually needs by taking little sips.

Lie Down in Shavasana: Shavasana is a simple yoga pose that requires lying on your back with your arms and legs relaxed and your palms facing up. While you're there, close your eyes and concentrate on each part of your body, from the toes to the head, one by one. Think positively about that area of your body, whether it be your knees or your navel, and notice how it feels right now. This is a fantastic technique to move energy from your body's overused areas to its unused ones. It helps ease tension and enhance focus.

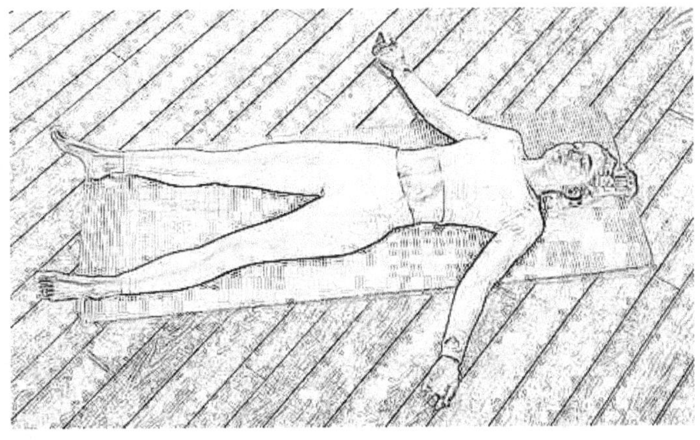

<u>*Do Dynamic Stretches*</u>: Dynamic stretches are exercises that involve several joints. As a result, they help increase blood circulation throughout your body and encourage coordination between your body's parts, which is exactly what you want to achieve before working out.

What are Reps and Sets?

The term "rep" stands for repetition in the context of exercise. It is a single exercise that has been executed. For instance, performing one push-up counts as performing one "rep" of a push-up. You completed 10 chest presses if you completed 10 reps of a chest press.

Sets are just groups of reps. For a particular exercise, you could perform a single set of reps or many sets. The routine of executing many sets is more prevalent, particularly if you want to increase your muscular strength or endurance.

For instance, you might perform three sets of 10 chest presses if your goal is to develop your chest muscles. This implies that after performing 10 chest presses, you rest briefly. After doing another 10 reps, you take another brief break. Then you do your final 10 repetitions before taking a little rest and then proceeding to your next workout.

Slow reps Vs Fast reps

How fast should you exercise?
The conventional wisdom is to go at a moderate tempo. Some might say that speed doesn't matter much, while others might

say going slow is definitely better. There are a few reasons why people want to slow down their reps. One of the goals is to increase the amount of time your muscles are under load. In the bodybuilding realm, this is known as Time Under Tension (TUT). The belief in these circles is that increasing TUT has underlying properties that improve growth. Mechanically, it might make sense since placing your fibers under longer tension should elicit greater fatigue and, thus, greater growth.

Slower reps can also restrict blood flow through longer contraction times. Cutting off blood circulation increases metabolite buildup within the working muscle, creating a bigger pump, and the occlusion also creates greater lactic acid buildup, which has been linked to muscle growth. Furthermore, slow rep believers have emphasized the importance of slowing down the negative portion of an exercise. This touches base with more growth theories where this negative, eccentric portion is responsible for greater muscle growth and even strength adaptation. One of which deals with eccentric contractions being responsible for the muscle tears during movement—that sore feeling you get after working out. Eccentric also activates recovery-induced satellite cells, cells that are pivotal for growth. Eccentric contractions have also been linked to the release of phosphatidic acid, which has also been linked to muscle growth.

However, studies that look directly at TUT have shown that, unfortunately, it doesn't provide any significant benefits. This is mainly because greater TUT means you have to use lighter weights. There are two things that generally dictate muscle growth effectiveness: One is making sure that you take your sets and reps as close as possible to 'Muscular Fatigue' or 'Muscular Failure'.

Studies have consistently shown the importance of volitional failure because failure means almost all muscle fibers are fully used. Slow and fast rep speeds will be able to achieve 'failure', but faster speeds have a small advantage. At a faster rep speed, you will not only be able to do a difficult workout but also simultaneously recruit more muscle fibers to exert a greater force. Slower reps also utilize mainly smaller Type 1 fibers, which don't help with growth as much as bigger Type 2 fibers. But even with that mentioned, reaching fatigue is the primary goal and is more important than the speed at which you get there. Along with reaching muscular fatigue, the other dictating factor is an increase in total work volume. Total work volume is the product of the number of reps, the number of sets, and the volume of weight. Studies consistently show that total work volume means greater muscle growth.

The effectiveness of slow rep training might be held back by the fact that, although it eventually recruits all your muscle fibers, it does not recruit as much simultaneously as faster reps would, which is important to muscle growth stimulation and also important to increasing muscle strength. Secondly, slower reps ultimately mean lower weights. Lower weight means lower total volume, and lower total volume means lower gains.

This doesn't mean slower reps are at all useless; as mentioned earlier, there are some merits to the hypothesis of eccentric contraction, but more importantly is the fact that, firstly, you are stronger during the eccentric, lowering phase of a movement, which adds more to your total work volume. An eccentric-focused set, commonly called 'Negatives' can serve as a finishing set to push your gains a bit farther. Another is that, by lifting a slower eccentric phase, you are ensuring that you are the one in control of your weight down instead of letting gravity do all the work, keeping more tension in your muscles. So, a generally slower rep scheme is good for beginners to work on form and prevent injury. Obviously, the faster you go, the less in control you are of the weight. By controlling your speed, you control the weight.

Rest between Sets

Some beginners ask the question, "How long do I wait before starting my next set?" According to the muscle growth research carried out by fitness expert Brad Schoenfeld, with more rest, you will be able to complete more reps, which is going to increase your total work volume. A higher total work volume will allow a higher dose-response for muscular and training adaptations.

Intensity is another factor to consider. If the program you are using doesn't push you close to muscular failure or the intensity of your exercise is a lot lower, then short rest can work just fine. In fact, there are benefits to using shorter rests with a lower load and a higher rep scheme since there will be a greater metabolic buildup of lactate, hydrogen ions, and inorganic phosphate, which have been observed to increase muscle growth signaling. On top of that, shorter rest intervals mean less time for the muscle to recover before lifting again, which can heighten motor unit recruitment and promote the development of the muscle pump.

Additionally, it has also been observed that longer rest intervals benefit multi-compound movements the most. Being that such exercises employ a high degree of muscle groups, total body fatigue can accumulate much quicker, thus requiring more rest.

So, while longer rest is good, shorter rest intervals do have a place when it comes to muscle growth too.

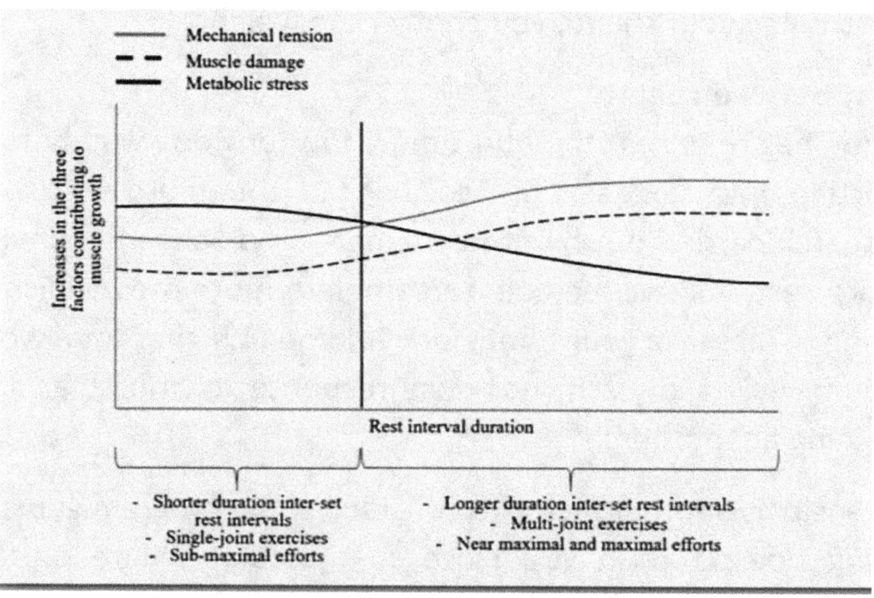

The hypothetical graphic above gives credence to deploying both rest intervals. As seen above, shorter rest hypothetically benefits growth by maintaining high levels of metabolic stress. Longer rest, on the other hand, can hypothetically benefit from a greater deal of mechanical tension and muscle damage from utilizing greater volumes and intensities.

In conclusion, if your goal is to completely maximize muscle hypertrophy, then you are best off deploying an inter-set rest interval between 1-3 minutes. But bear in mind that the benefit isn't all that substantial compared to using less rest, and you also need to consider that resting more will increase the total duration of your entire session. If you can only muster 45 minutes to an hour of workout time, then a shorter rest interval would be suitable for you. The researchers advise spending the first part of your session on multi-joint heavy movements, i.e., triceps dips, while using longer rests. After that, you can focus on isolation single-joint exercises, i.e., squats, with shorter rests.

Common Muscle-Building Mistake

Not Training Close to Failure

To build muscle, the goal is actually to activate and fatigue them in order to drive the mechanism of muscle hypertrophy adaptation. First, ensure that you are maximizing motor unit recruitment, where the size principle dictates that higher threshold muscle fibers, like Type 2 fibers, are only recruited once fatigue-resistant fibers, like Type 1, reach muscular fatigue.

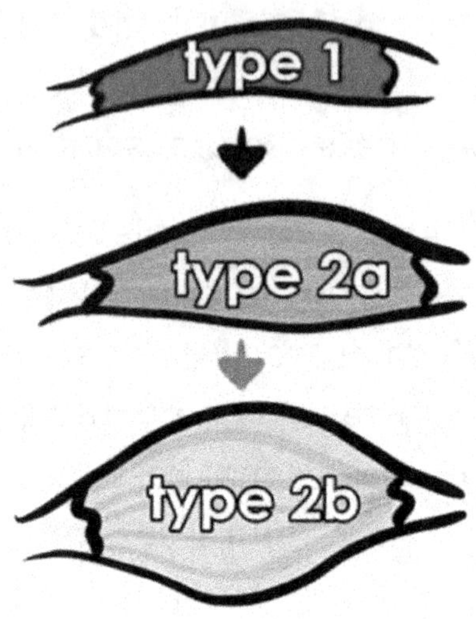

In short, the best means to fatigue and activate all muscle fibers is to train with relatively high effort, often achieved by training close to failure. The only issue, however, is that people's perception of failure is often a bit off. Or rather, many people think they are training close to failure when they actually have plenty left in their tank. In order to deal with this inaccuracy, occasionally train to actual failure, the point at which you cannot concentrically move your weight without sacrificing form.

Experiencing actual failure safely will help you understand when to stop short of failure in future workouts. In many programs, it is recommended to train to the point where you have about 1 to 2 reps in reserve (RIR). This simply means that had you continued your set, you would only muster 1 to 2 reps before reaching 'failure'. As mentioned, reaching this point consistently will ensure that all muscle fibers are properly activated, giving your muscle the best stimulus for growth.

Mismanaging Progression and Volume

Progressing in volume is vital in your training, especially if your goal is to build muscle. According to studies, the best predictor of muscle hypertrophy is, in fact, volume, which is commonly measured as Reps x Sets x Load. However, this doesn't mean that more and more volume will always produce more and more gains. As a matter of fact, too much volume is shown to have diminishing returns, to the point of curtailing adaptation. The big question that is still up for debate is: At what point is more volume no longer effective?' A simple explanation of this is that it is a reactionary approach that gauges how one responds to volume progression. How you respond to a certain amount of volume and how it affects your gains, strength and effort level, recovery, and mood should then reflect your progression programming. If you are getting sufficient gains from something like 12 sets per muscle group and dialing that up to 15 sets doesn't make things better or even worse, then simply maintaining 12 sets might be best.

This is not to disregard the place of volume in building muscle. The main takeaway is to progress your volume appropriately based on your actual results instead of trying to push more volume in order to see results. Results dictate progression, not progression.

Cutting When You Need to Build

A lot of people, ironically those with little to no workout experience, think that burning fat is the missing ingredient to their muscle aesthetic. The problem lies, however, when people overemphasize fat burning to the point where they start eating so little that the nutrients become insufficient to support continuous and optimal muscle growth. Even if burning fat is your main goal, preserving lean mass should still be a priority. That is best achieved with a slight calorie deficit paired with both cardio and resistance training.

For most people who are carrying an average amount of weight and fat, the better approach will be to stick to a decent training program, shoot for more protein and healthy whole food choices, and stay close to your calorie maintenance—the number of calories sufficient for you to sustain your current weight. It is amazing how just sticking to these fundamentals plus getting enough sleep would get people much closer to their aesthetic goals than just burning fat. Instead of reducing body fat percentage by reducing fat mass, increasing the lean mass to fat ratio is much more ideal. Again, it is important to stick to the fundamentals and let the result come to you. And finally, stay consistent.

CHAPTER TWO
BEGINNER'S CALISTHENICS CATEGORIES

When it has to do with calisthenics, irrespective of your fitness level, you should endeavor to learn the basics, also referred to as the fundamentals. These serve as the foundation for the growth of your strength. It may be broken down into several parts:

Push Exercises

Pushing exercises work a variety of body parts, including the arms, core, hips, legs, and chest. They come in a variety of forms, such as push-ups, squats, and shoulder presses. By implementing these into your training program, you will receive several benefits for your mental and physical health and overall quality of life. Pushing exercises can be used to strengthen your body and increase its functionality for everyday tasks. Pushups and other muscle-building activities help support the structure of your body, which enhances the health of your bones. Pushing exercises use a variety of muscles, which means your heart will have to work harder to circulate blood throughout your body. By accelerating your heart rate and working your aerobic system, these exercises can also help you lose weight. Below are some of the push exercises for beginners.

Push-Ups

Push-ups are one of the most fundamental bodyweight exercises and are very popular. The movement is simple, can be done everywhere, and is very effective because you are using a lot of muscles at the same time. The problem is that a lot of people concentrate on quantity instead of quality when doing push-ups. To avoid this, focus on these vital points to make your push-up perfect.

<u>Body Position</u>: A push-up is not only a triceps, chest, and shoulder movement. Most people neglect the tension in the abdominal muscles, the hips, and the legs. Often, they form an arched back and lack body tension. To avoid this, tilt your pelvis backward and keep your buttocks squeezed tight.

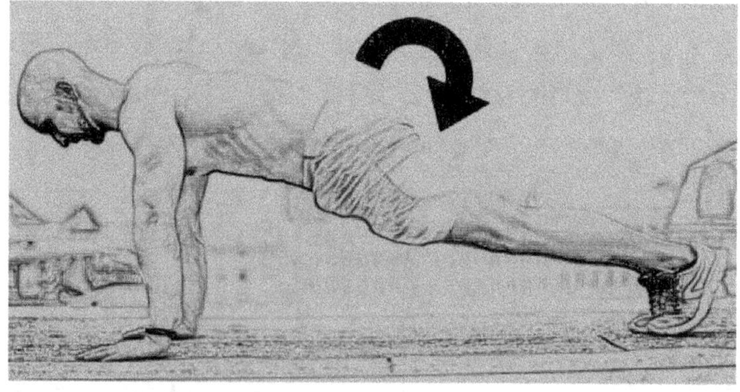

The movement gets a lot harder with this, but it is also much more effective.

<u>Arm Position</u>: The arm position doesn't really matter in terms of perfect execution. A perfect push-up can be done with a wide or narrow hand placement.

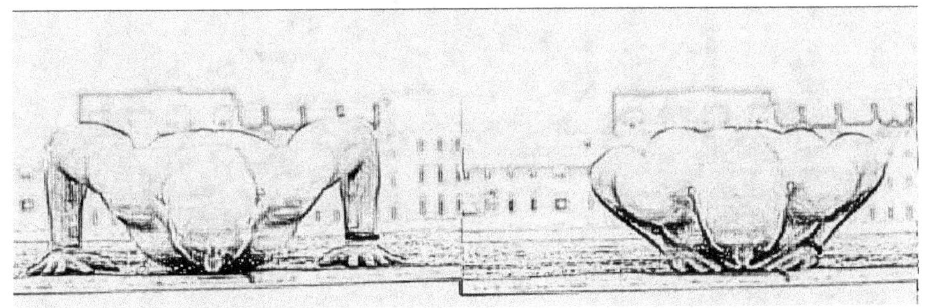

But it is important to place your wrist in a nearly vertical line under your shoulder when you do the standard push-up.

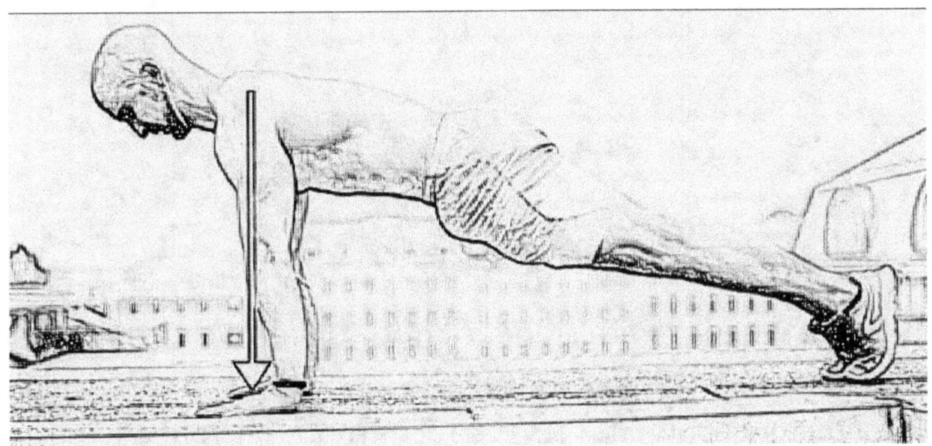

Although this rule still has some exceptions, one of which is the pseudo-planche push-up, which puts the focus more on your shoulders.

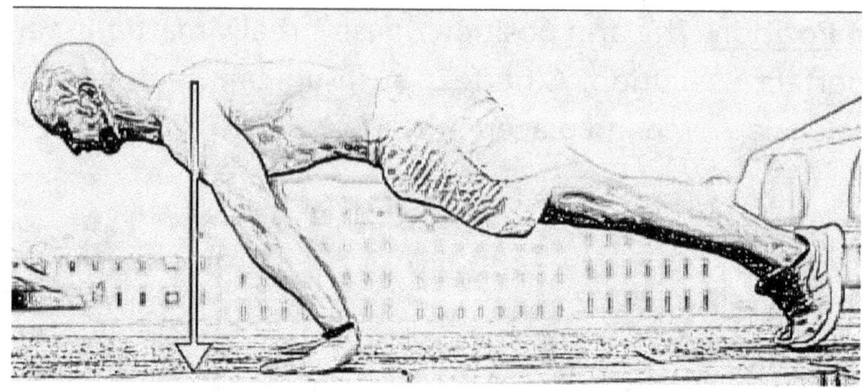

Or when you are doing splinx push-ups, which are a triceps-dominant movement.

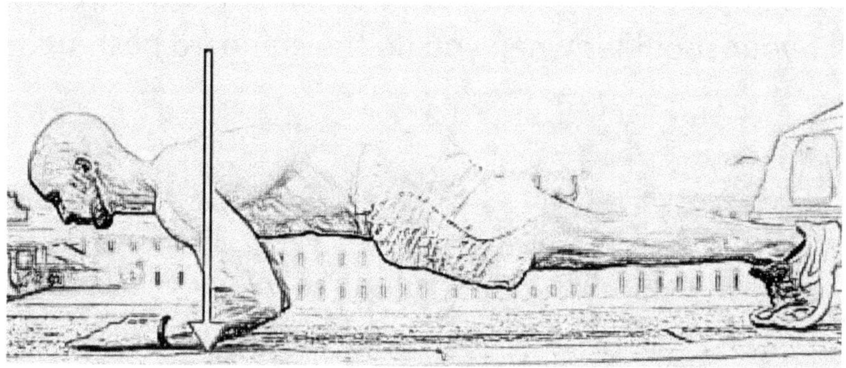

If you are working with standard push-ups and choose a wide grip, it involves the chest more than a close hand placement. And a hand placement sets the focus more on your triceps.

<u>Range of Motion</u>: This is quite simple; however, don't cheat. Go all the way up and all the way down. And let your body straighten up. Don't decrease the range of motion by bringing your head forward or your hips down.

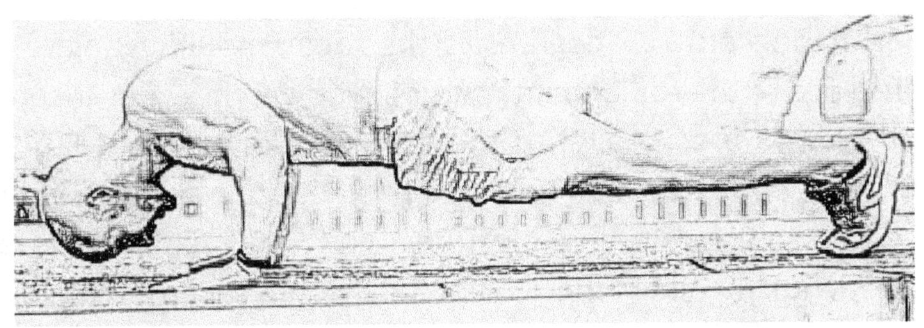

<u>Shoulder blade Movement</u>: This is a very neglected point. When you are going down, your shoulder blades come together, and when you are going up, they go apart.

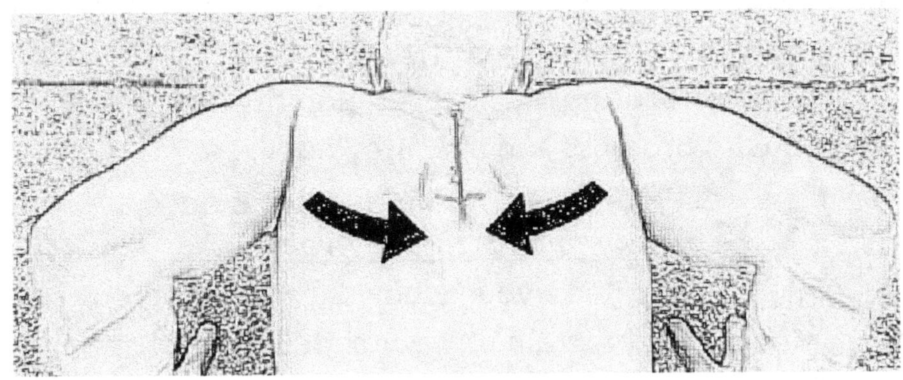

You should also focus on pushing them downward instead of upward. If you are too weak in the shoulder girdle, your shoulder blades come together because you are not able to hold your body against gravity. This can be especially seen at the top of the movement. When you are going down, always focus on the tension and an active shoulder blade; don't let yourself fall into your structures.

Throughout the entire push-up, keep the core engaged. Taking a deep breath, carefully lower your chest toward the floor while keeping your elbows bent and tucked in rather than flaring out. 45 degrees is the ideal shoulder angle in reference to the torso. Continue going down until your triceps and elbows are parallel to the ground. Exhale when lifting your body off the ground. As you push back up through your hands to the starting posture, you will experience a contraction in your chest, shoulders, and triceps muscles. Before performing this motion again, make sure you have completed the range of motion by going all the way up and locking your arms out.

With these points listed, although it might be much harder to do and your maximum repetition will drop, that shouldn't matter. Always focus on quality over quantity. And you will be rewarded with progress and a healthy body.

Common Errors to Avoid

Out-Flared Elbows: Keep your elbows from flaring out since doing so puts a lot of strain on your shoulders and can cause injury. According to studies, flared elbows result in less chest and triceps activation as well as decreased strength and power gains because of the restricted range of motion. The closer you place your arm to the body, the more your elbows point backward. The wider you place your arms, the more your elbows go away from your body, but they are still more backward than to the side.

To avoid this, use a little wider hand placement than a narrow hand placement and tuck your elbows in at a 45-degree angle instead of flaring them out.

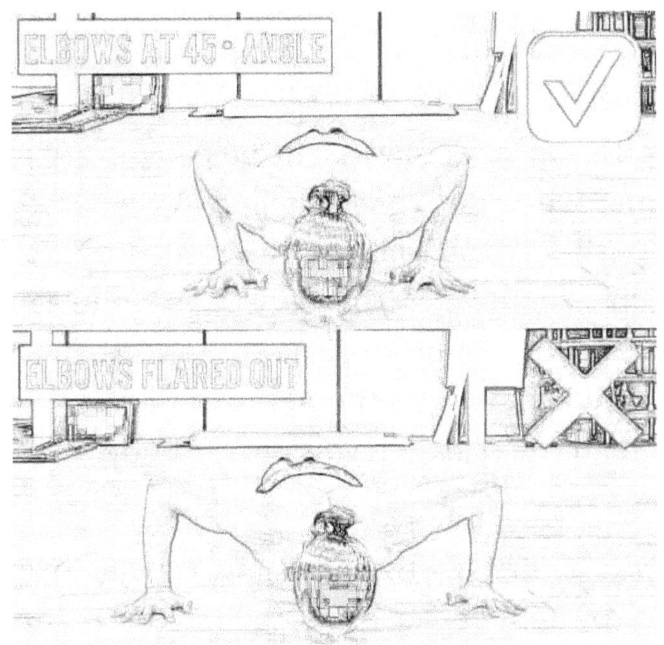

No Body Tension: People frequently have arched backs and a lack of bodily tension. They adopt poor posture as a result, with their backs arching and their hips sagging. When the glutes and core are not fully engaged, it happens. To correct this, concentrate on keeping your lower back flat throughout this action by using your core and glutes simultaneously. This will help to strengthen your core and ensure proper form. When practicing this exercise, you can check your form by filming yourself or glancing in the mirror.

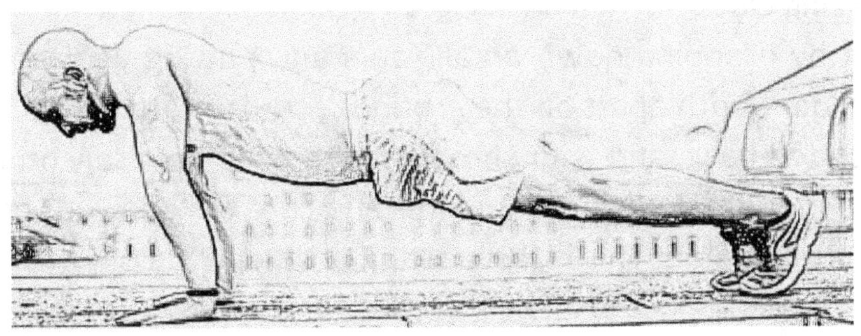

Knee push-up

The knee push-up is a bodyweight pushing exercise that will help you improve upper body strength in preparation for the complete push-up. You will get the same results from this form of regression exercise because it uses the same sets of muscles and follows the same motion as a regular push-up. Since you'll be kneeling, as the name implies, the action will be simpler, and the strain on your upper body muscles will be reduced.

Push-ups are a terrific strengthening activity to practice if you're new to them because they build your triceps muscles and chest. The knee push-up is an excellent workout for beginners who wish to strengthen their triceps and chest muscles. They are relatively easy because you are pushing less of your body weight while you are on your knees as opposed to your toes. Simply put, performing knee push-ups places less strain on the upper-body muscles. Knee push-ups are a fantastic alternative to standard push-ups for the purpose of developing shoulder, chest, and arm strength while also strengthening the core muscles.

<u>Working Out</u>

Start by dropping down on all fours and putting your hands shoulder-width apart on the ground. Your legs are joined and extended back, and your shoulders are piled precisely on top of your wrists. Engage your glutes and core to keep your body in a straight line. This is the starting position.

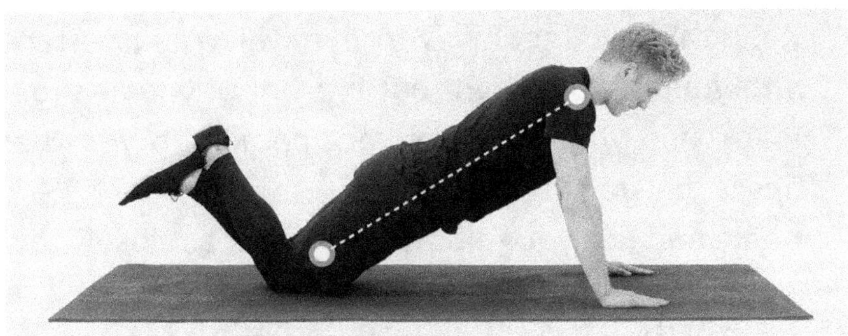

Inhale deeply as you push your chest downward until your elbows are roughly at a 90-degree angle. Instead of flaring out, your elbows are brought in towards your chest. Throughout the entire movement, keep your core engaged.

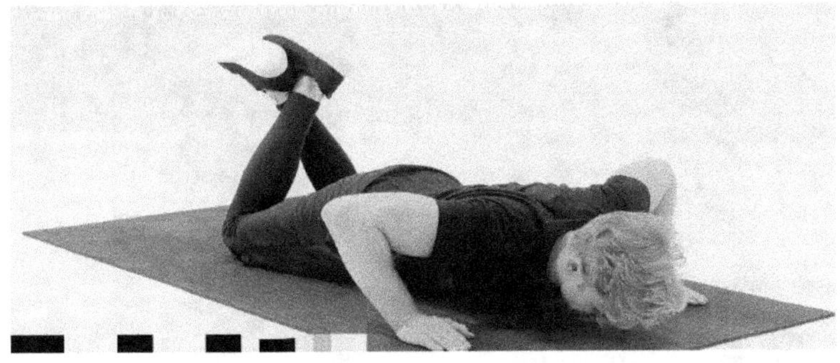

As you push yourself back up to your starting posture, exhale through your mouth. At the highest position, tighten your triceps, abs, and chest. To guarantee a broad range of motion, lock both arms fully out before repeating.

Wall Push Up

Push-ups against a wall work your shoulders, back, triceps, and chest. If you are unable to perform knee push-ups at this time, this exercise is an excellent place to start because it puts more of the weight on the feet than the upper body. The steps are as follows:

1. Stand tall, two feet away from a wall. You are standing with your arms straight out in front of you at shoulder width, and your shoulders are parallel to your hands. This is the starting posture.
2. Inhale and flex your elbows as you tilt as closely toward the wall as you can. Consider moving your feet closer to the wall if you feel like you're stretching too far.
3. Exhale and push yourself back to the starting posture.

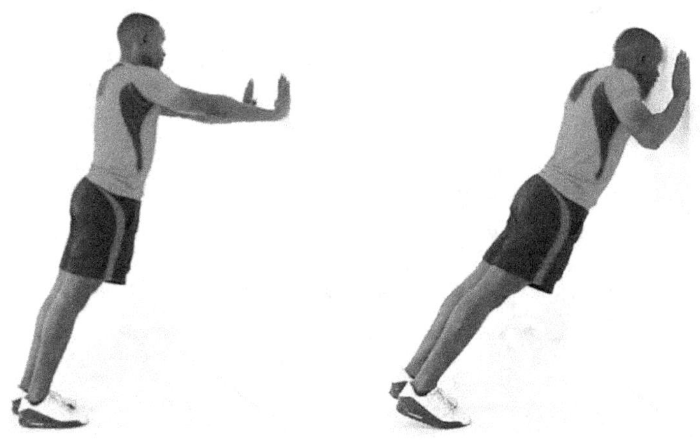

To focus on various muscle groups and parts of the muscle, you might experiment with different hand placements. The shoulder-width grip works on your triceps and middle chest. The diamond grip will isolate the triceps and reduce chest involvement. The wide grip puts pressure on the back, shoulders, and outer chest.

Incline Push-Up

The incline push-up is a fantastic body-weight pushing exercise for the lower chest region. As your hands will be on something higher, there will be less strain on your upper body than with a regular push-up. In an incline position, the legs carry the majority of your weight. Men's Health recommends that if you want to improve at push-ups, you should perform incline push-ups rather than knee push-ups to develop true strength as you progress toward a full push-up. This is due to the fact that knee push-ups do not appropriately educate the core and glutes to stabilize the body. Incline push-ups are ideal for beginners since they help improve the endurance and strength needed for standard push-ups.

Begin by standing tall in front of an elevated surface, like a plyometric box or a bench. Place both hands shoulder-width apart on the edge of the bench. You have your feet together and your arms outstretched. Engage your core and glutes to keep your body upright. This is the startup position.

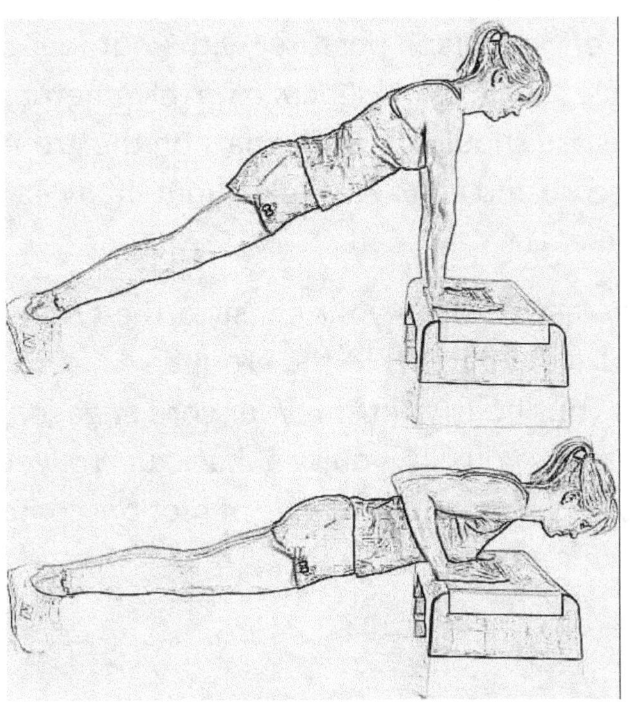

While performing incline push-ups, you can adjust your grip position to target various areas of the muscles being used. This would be more convenient than executing them on the floor. Diamond push-ups, for example, target the triceps, while broad push-ups target the outside chest. Exhale as you push yourself away from the platform to get back into your starting position. To guarantee a full range of motion, lock both arms out before repeating the rep.

Decline Push-Up

Decline push-ups are the opposite of uphill push-ups. It is done with your feet on an elevated surface and both hands on the ground, putting extra strain on the upper-body muscles. This version focuses on the upper chest and anterior deltoids. The steps are as follows:

1. Start off in a plank posture, with your feet on a raised surface, such as a bench or a plyometric box. Your hands are shoulder-width apart on the ground. Engage your core and glutes to keep your body in a straight line.

2. Inhale as you drop your chest to the ground, bringing your triceps parallel to the ground.
Keep your body rigid and your core engaged.
3. Exhale as you lift yourself back up to your starting posture. For complete range of motion, completely lock out your arms.

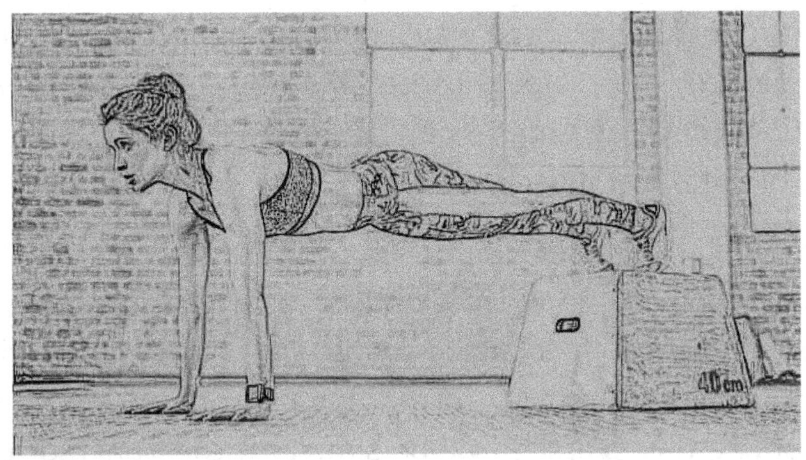

Triceps Dip

The dip, commonly referred to as triceps dips, is an upper-body complex exercise that strengthens the triceps, shoulders, and chest. This is one of the essential calisthenics exercises that you should learn to master since it will improve your pushing strength, allowing you to perform more push-up repetitions, as well as your transitional strength for powerful maneuvers like the muscle-up.

Without using a gym membership or any expensive equipment, dips can provide you with superb chest and triceps exercises. Chair dips can be done in the comfort of your own home using chairs, and you can even increase the difficulty by performing dips on a straight bar or a parallel bar. Our triceps muscles allow us to extend our elbows, and they are also powerful forearm extenders. Pushing with the triceps is a common movement that is employed in daily tasks including opening doors, plugging things into outlets, and moving furniture across a room.

Dips can be done in three ways: bench dips, straight bar dips, and parallel bar dips. These methods include several variations, such as progressions, regressions, and grips, that focus on different muscle areas.

Bench Dips

Bench dips, commonly referred to as chair dips, are the easiest and most feasible form of dip exercise, with three progressions within this form alone. Keep in mind that performing this exercise will be simpler if the bench or chair is higher. To accomplish this, you must:

1. Place both hands on a bench or other raised surface. Your arms should be fully extended, and the tips of your fingertips should be facing forward. Fully extend your legs while maintaining a strong core. This is the starting posture.
2. Inhale while bending your elbows until your triceps are level with the ground and lowering your torso gradually. Maintain a strong core and straight legs.
3. Exhale as you extend both arms and push through your palms to return to the initial posture.

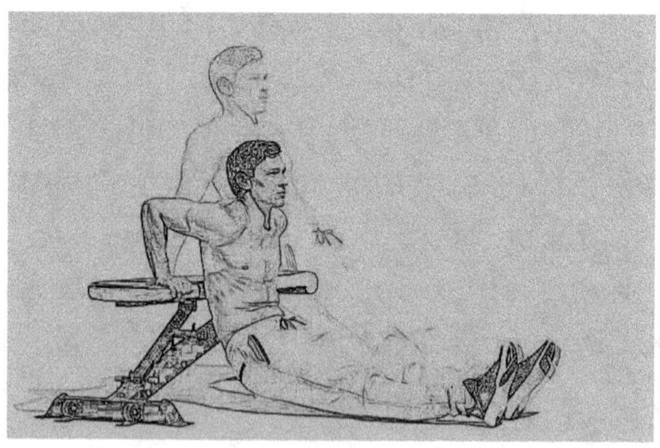

The pressure on the upper body can be reduced by bending the knees in the starting position, and you can progress by setting your feet upon an elevated platform that is level with your palms. Furthermore, performing dips with a wider grip or with the elbows flaring forth will emphasize the chest muscles more than doing them with the elbows pointing inside, which will emphasize the triceps more.

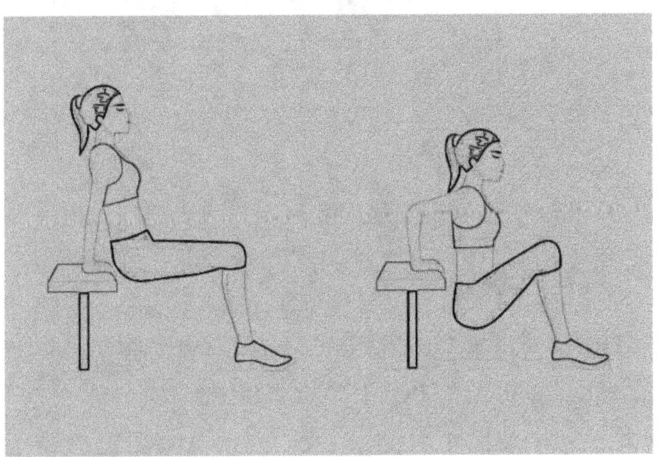

Parallel Dips

Parallel dips are a continuation of bench dips in that your feet are lifted off the floor, putting extra strain on the upper body's muscles. To do this, you will:

1. Place both hands on parallel bars, with your arms locked out by your sides. Bend your knees slightly and elevate your feet off the floor behind you. Maintain a firm core and an upright torso. This is the starting posture.

2. Inhale as you bend your elbows and lower your body. Lower yourself until your elbows form a 90-degree angle. Ensure your core and legs are engaged all through this movement.

3. Exhale as you return to the beginning position, fully locking both arms out to provide a full circle of motion.

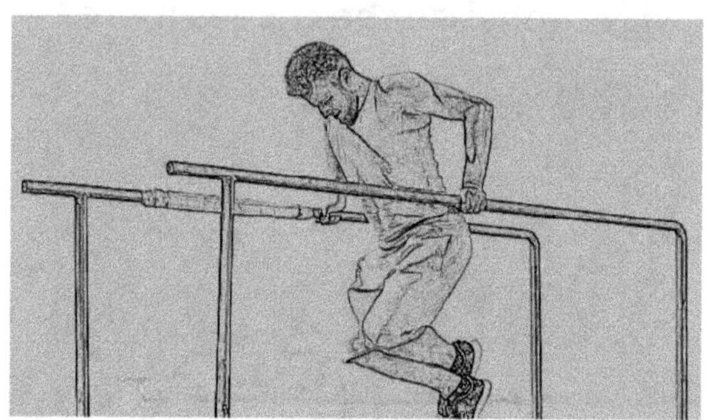

If you are still unable to perform parallel dips well, you can regress by putting your feet down to lessen the strain on your upper body. Begin with one leg on the ground, then progress to lifting both of your legs off the ground as you gain strength. Resistance bands are another way to increase strength for full dips. Place a band over the parallel bars and place your knees on top to ease the pressure off the targeted muscles.

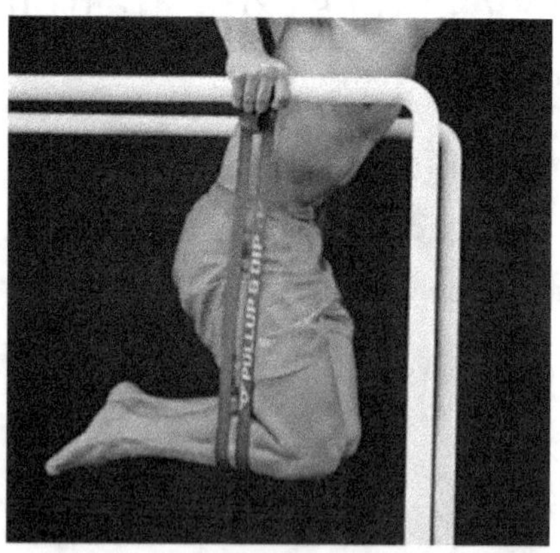

To target various points on the muscle, you can change the parallel bars' width. For instance, targeting the outer upper chest will be accomplished by turning both hands inside. The lower chest area will be targeted if you place your hands in an inverted grip while externally spinning them outward.

Straight Bar Dips

The arm and shoulder positions make this version more difficult than parallel bar dips since they emphasize the chest muscles more. Additionally, because you have to move your body around the bar, it calls for more core engagement. If you want to accomplish a muscle-up, it is highly advised that you perfect this exercise. To accomplish this, you must:

1. With your hands shoulder-width apart and pronated, hold a straight bar in place. Keep your feet together and contract your glutes, quadriceps, and core. This is the starting posture.
2. Inhale while bending your elbows to lower your body into a dip. In order to balance yourself, lean over the bar and stretch your legs slightly forward while keeping your feet close together. Throughout this action, your core remains tight. Try to touch the bar with your lower chest.
3. Breathe out as you raise yourself back up to the beginning position by extending your arms.

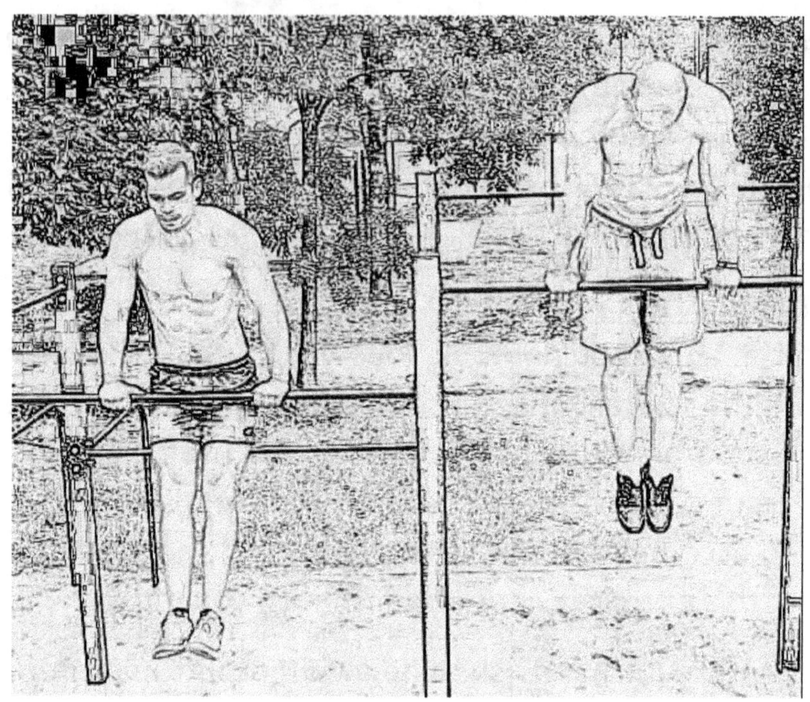

Straight bar dips are fantastic because you can adjust your hand placement to target various angles within a muscle as well as various muscle groups. You can alternate between a pronated or supinated grip with a short, shoulder-width, wide grip.

Pull Exercises

Pulling exercises are motions used in strength training that entail contracting muscles to pull weight inward toward the body. The biceps, hamstrings, trapezius, obliques, and all of one's back muscles are the main muscles used in a pull workout.

A combination of fundamental exercises that incorporate both pulling and pushing motions should be part of your training program if you want to be well-rounded. The following are just a few of the many advantages of pull exercises:

- Strengthens back muscles, arms, and legs. Regular back exercises can help you loosen up your back muscles, which improves mobility and lowers your risk of injury and back pain. Additionally, developing back strength is beneficial for sports-related movements like rowing, paddling, and swimming the breaststroke, as well as necessary daily actions like properly lifting an object off the ground.
- Increases strength and burns calories. Pulling exercises are a terrific strength training technique that, for instance, burns roughly 1 calorie per pull-up, despite the fact that you could be better off performing a cardiovascular activity if your aim is to burn an excessive amount of calories.
- Improves mental health. Researchers found that resistance training exercisers with mild to moderate depression experienced a substantial improvement after performing these exercises a few days per week.

Standard Pull-Up

One of the most basic calisthenics exercises for developing upper-body strength and endurance is the pull-up. It is frequently used as a physical exam in settings ranging from schools to the military. Pull-ups are one of the most effective exercises for developing a bigger, stronger back. As a result, many players from various sports utilize them in their training.

Once you master this exercise, it will benefit other fantastic skills you learn, like one-arm pull-ups, muscle-ups, back levers, and front levers. This single exercise will kickstart your calisthenics journey. The pull-up is an intermediate-level exercise, as you have to lift your body weight vertically, putting the majority of the strain on your lats. To be able to maintain stability while performing this exercise, one needs to have intermediate-level core strength.

<u>Working Out</u>

Hold the bar with both palms facing forward and approximately shoulder-width apart. Put your thumbs beneath and around the bar while you hold it firmly. Your legs should be close together or crossed, and both arms should be completely extended.

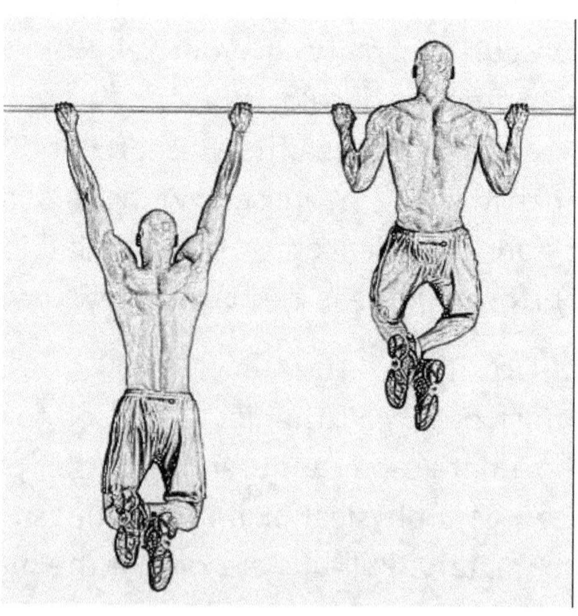

Maintain a strong grip on your legs and core at all times. These muscles will serve as your stabilizers, giving you better control over your entire body during pull-ups.

Still hanging, take a breath in through your mouth, then let it out as you draw yourself up by bending your elbows and dragging your arms downward. Pull yourself up so that your chin is over the bar. The lats and biceps will be the primary musclesd being worked. Maintain your core engagement during this movement. Your shoulders must be lowered and your scapulars retracted during the motion.

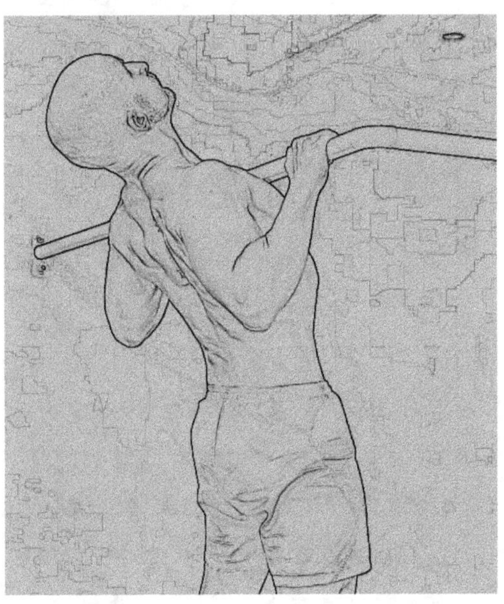

Inhale as you lower yourself to your starting posture with your arms fully locked out. This guarantees an entire range of motion, which will engage multiple muscles and improve a pull-up's overall effectiveness. Maintaining a broad range of motion will ensure that your efforts are not in vain.

As a beginner, the pull-up is one exercise you should slowly add to your training regimen, as it will be worthwhile in the long run and help you get better at other exercises.

Chin Up

The chin-up is an intensive body-weight pulling exercise that strengthens and expands the arms, especially the biceps, latissimus dorsi, and posterior deltoids. A supinated grip is used in chin-ups, which will emphasize the biceps more.

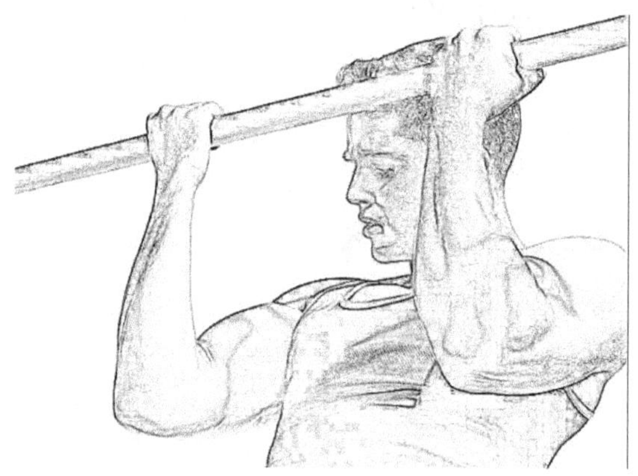

The American Council on Exercise claims that chin-ups can strengthen the muscles that support the spine and help with posture, appearance, and grip strength. This is an intermediate-advanced level workout since you must lift your entire body weight using only your upper body muscles. If you weigh 150 pounds, you are lifting 150 pounds, and 200 pounds is the same. Beginners shouldn't lose heart because training will be worthwhile regardless of the effort they put forth.

<u>Working Out</u>

Grab the bar in a supinated or underhand grip with your hands towards you and about shoulder-width apart. Your thumbs should encircle the bar from underneath. Your feet are close together, and both arms are fully stretched. This is the starting position.

Draw your belly button nearer your spine to tighten your core. You'll be able to regulate your body better and engage your core as a result. Exhale as you raise yourself up by bending your elbows, bringing your arms downward, and constricting your shoulder blades. Maintain a firm core the entire time you pull yourself up until your chin is over the bar. The biceps and lats are where you will feel the most involvement.

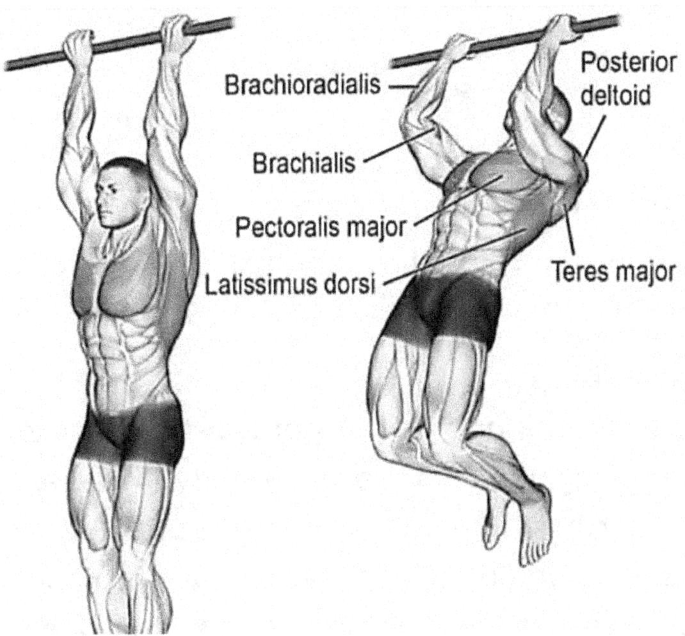

You can experiment with various grip configurations, such as close grip and wide grip. As a result, various muscle groups will be isolated. Your biceps will be targeted with a thin grip.

Your lats will be targeted with a wide hold, while your middle back will be targeted with a grip at shoulder width.

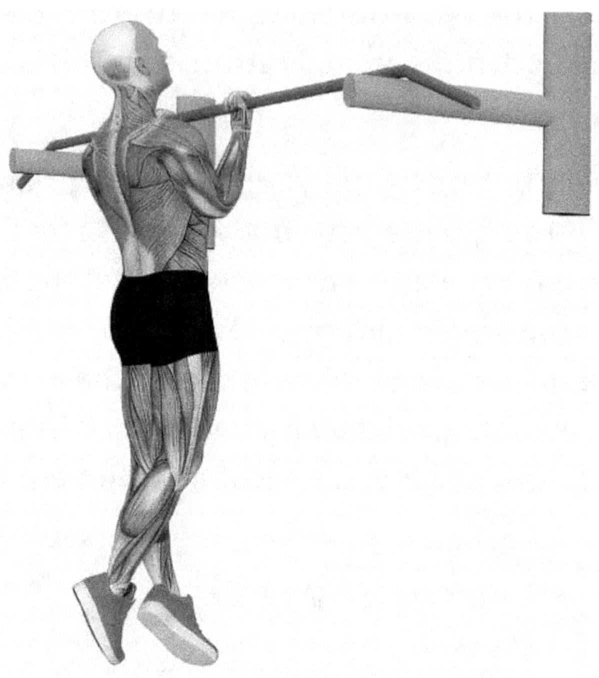

Inhale softly through the nostrils as you return to the starting posture. To achieve a thorough range of motion, fully extend both arms before repeating the rep.

Australian Pull-up
The Australian pull-up is a form of calisthenics exercise that enhances pulling power in the upper body. This is excellent for beginners because it serves as a warm-up exercise for pull-ups. Since you would have to lie beneath the bar with your arms extended and heels on the ground, your body would be on an inclined slope, using less body weight. However, this exercise follows the same motion pattern as the pull-up, which will strengthen your arms, shoulders, and back.

The Australian pull-up targets the latissimus dorsi, biceps, abdominal muscles, rear deltoids, and forearm muscles in the upper body. In order to help support the body, certain muscles in the lower body, including the hamstrings, quadriceps, and glutes, must be engaged.

<u>Working Out</u>

Body position: Position yourself beneath a low bar with both hands shoulder-width apart and your arms straight. When pulling up, align your shoulders with the bar so that your center chest meets it. Straighten your body by keeping your feet together and engaging your glutes and quads to keep your body taut. Your body ought to be positioned on an incline.

Tightly grip the bar: There are many grip variations you can do to perform this exercise, but for now, you would have a tight, pronated grip, shoulders width apart, with your thumbs underneath the bar. Stay in an active hang with your scapulars retracted, as this will provide you with additional support for the shoulder and increase power and muscle mass.

Pull to chest: Exhale while you pull the bar directly to your chest, contracting your biceps and rear deltoids while you maintain a straight line with your torso. You should experience resistance in both the lower body muscles, such as the glutes, quadriceps, and hamstrings, as well as the upper body muscular groups, such as the upper back, shoulders, chest, and arms.

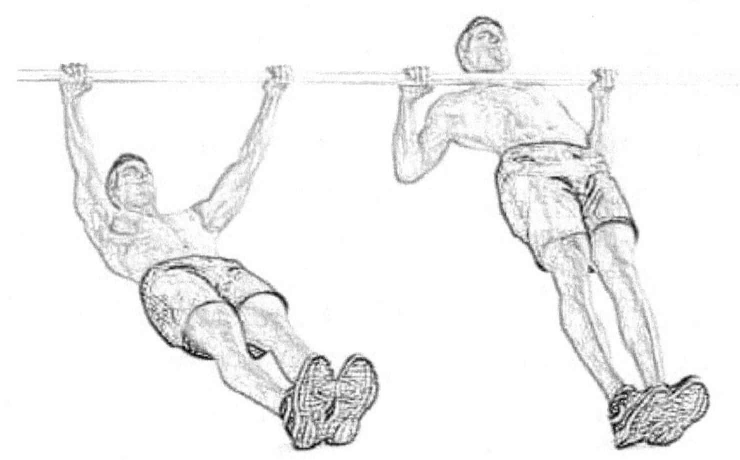

Retract your scapula: To boost muscle contraction and strengthen your shoulder blades, bring your shoulder blades together as you pull yourself up. This is known as retracting your scapula. In addition to this, it will help you develop stable joints, effective arm movement, and better posture.

Return to the starting position: Inhale as you descend towards the beginning position, lock both elbows out, and then raise yourself back up. By preserving a full range of motion, this improves muscle balance, joint stability, appropriate activation of working muscles, and movement quality as a whole.

The Australian pull-up as a progression is very important for improving your pull-ups, strengthening them, and increasing total repetitions. Similar muscle groups to those used in pull-ups are worked out. They're an excellent way to develop the upper back, shoulders, arms, and core muscles. You get better at isolating and using the muscles that move your body vertically upward toward the bar above you with every repetition you perform. Australian pull-ups are an excellent addition to your back-to-school workouts because they'll help you get stronger and advance you closer to a pull-up.

Dead Hanging

Dead hanging is a wonderful exercise in which you simply hang from a pull-up bar with your feet lifted off the ground, using either a pronated or supinated grip. There won't be any action, pulling, or pushing while you do this workout. Dead hangings go beyond simply hanging. It has numerous health advantages for your body, including spinal decompression and increased grip power.

Despite being simple, deadlifts are incredibly good for your body because they train a variety of muscle groups. The forearms, hand and wrist flexors, latissimus dorsi, trapezius, anterior and posterior deltoids, and abdominals are the muscles targeted.

<u>Working Out</u>
1. Start by putting yourself under a safe bar. You can step onto a bench or other elevated surface to reach the bar with your hands.
2. Hold the bar tightly with a pronated or overhand grip, shoulder-width apart. Your thumbs should encircle the bar from underneath.
3. With your feet off the ground and your body hanging from the bar in a straight line, lock your arms out. Maintain a straight posture with your shoulders raised and avoid bending your arms; such hang is passive.

4. Hold for 10–60 seconds, and then repeat for 4 sets.

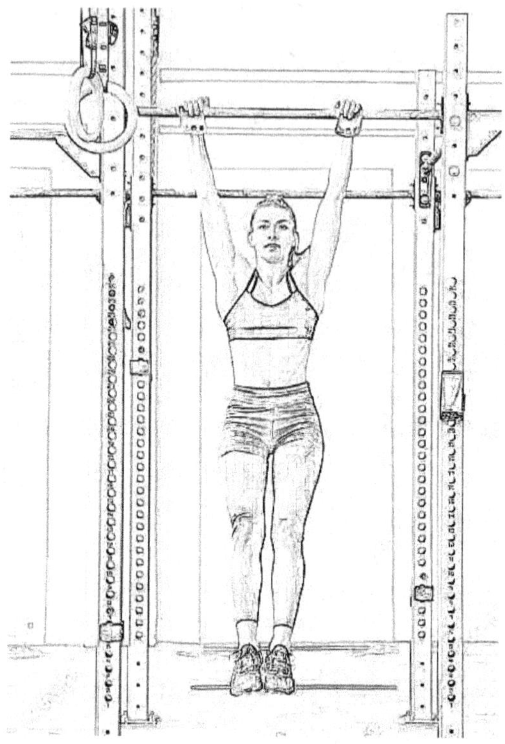

Harder variations of this exercise involve you using an object to hang on to or changing your hand position (supinated, use of rings and towels, single arm, mixed grip).

Core Exercise

A core exercise is any exercise that requires you to coordinate the use of your back and abdominal muscles. For instance, utilizing free weights in a way that requires maintaining a steady trunk can train and build a number of your muscles, including your core muscles. Integrating core movements into your fitness program has positive emotional and physical effects. Core workouts target the muscles in your pelvis, hips, lower back, and abdomen. Together, these muscles can be worked to improve stability and balance. Improved balance and stability mean fewer injuries. Almost every workout done in calisthenics involves having a strong core, thus making core exercise an important regimen for every beginner.

Performing daily activities like bending over to tie a shoe, sitting in a chair, or ascending stairs can all be made easier by having a strong core. Simple everyday movements like this grow more difficult as we age, which is why it's critical to have a healthy lifestyle and follow a decent fitness regimen that includes a variety of fundamental exercises, including core workouts.

Leg Raises

Leg raises are a powerful strength-training exercise that helps shape six-pack abs and develop a rock-solid core. Although there are several variations to this exercise, ranging in difficulty from beginner to advanced, the lying leg Lifts will be the main exercise we concentrate on. The only thing you need for this is a comfortable floor on which to lie down. This workout targets the rectus abdominis, particularly the lower abs, as well as other muscle groups throughout your body. As the muscles in the abdomen are used isometrically to support the body throughout the motion, it also targets the hip flexors as well as the quadriceps and the obliques.

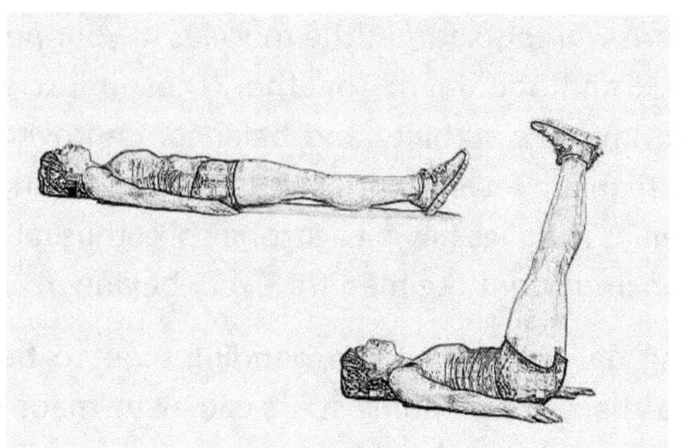

<u>Working Out</u>

1. To begin, lie flat on the ground with your legs straight out in front of you. To stabilize your body, keep both feet together and place your hands by your sides. You should always keep your toes pointed. For support and comfort, use a yoga mat, an exercise mat, or a carpet.

2. To prevent arching, use your core and glutes to drive your lower back flat on the ground. If you can't maintain your lower back flat or are having pain there, place your palms beneath your buttocks or a cloth beneath your lower back.

3. Inhale, then let it out as you raise your legs all the way up to the sky until your buttocks rise off the floor, keeping your legs straight up and toes pointed. Your torso and legs ought to form a 90-degree angle. There should be no space between your lower back and the ground, so make sure to contract your abs to force your lower back into the ground. By doing so, you can protect your spine while working on your abdominal muscles.

4. Take a deep breath and lower your legs until they are two to three inches above the ground. The idea is to go as close to the ground as you can without touching it. Refuse to be ruled by gravity. Your breathing technique—exhaling as you raise your arms and inhaling when you lower them—is what matters most. You'll be able to complete more repetitions while exerting less effort.

Common variations on this exercise include:

Side Leg Raises: This version is also suitable for beginners because of its ease of execution. It targets a variety of muscles, including the inner thighs, glutes, obliques, and abdominals. You would lay on your side with your feet and hips piled on top of one another to execute this. Your right hand is supporting your head while your legs are extended straight ahead. Lift your upper leg carefully until you can feel your hips tilting upward while maintaining core stability.

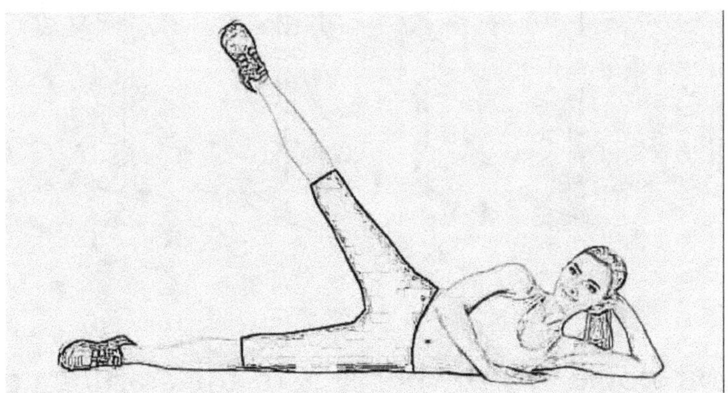

Avoid rotating your hips either forward or backward, and keep them stable and looking forward. After a little pause, bring your leg back down to the starting posture. After completing the prescribed number of reps, switch sides and perform the same number of reps on the new side.

Hanging Leg Raises: This is an intermediate-level workout because it takes strength in the upper body to hang from a bar. The abdominals, hip flexors, obliques, and quadriceps are the muscles that are worked, as are supporting muscles like the lats and forearms. You will require a pull-up bar just above you that you can jump onto and grab firmly with your shoulders spread apart in order to complete the hanging leg raises. Keep your feet together, your toes pointed, and your body straight. Keep your legs straight as you raise them until they form a 90-degree angle with your body. As you raise yourself, feel the abdominal muscles contract.

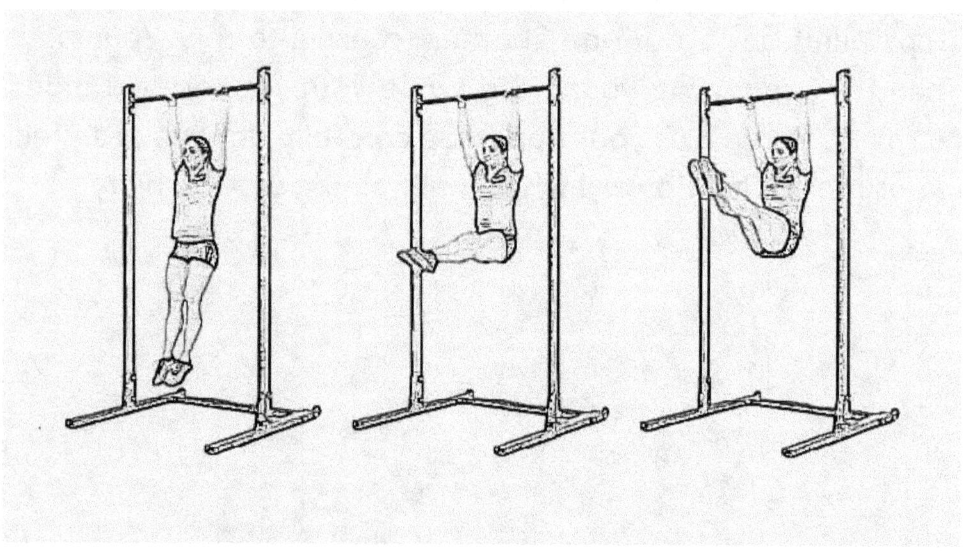

Lastly, you would return your legs to the starting point and concentrate on engaging your core to lessen the swing of your torso.

Mountain Climber

Mountain climbers are a powerful bodyweight workout that emphasizes the arms, core, shoulders, and quadriceps in particular. This exercise requires you to start in a plank posture and alternate between bringing a knee to your chest and bringing it back out. This exercise contains a cardio component that will increase your muscle endurance. Although they may appear simple, mountain climbers will increase your heart rate, burn calories, and help you develop a stronger core. You can perform this exercise wherever is most convenient for you, such as at home, in your office, in a hotel room, or in a parking lot.

Research shows that core strength exercises are more beneficial than traditional resistance exercises for reducing persistent low back pain. Furthermore, there are various bodyweight variations available, and people can freely do core workouts at home without any specific equipment. The mountain climbers target both upper- and lower-body muscles simultaneously, giving you a full-body workout. The glutes, abdominals, and hip flexors are the main muscles engaged. The anterior deltoids, hamstrings, quadriceps, triceps, and calves are the secondary muscles that are exercised.

Mountain Climber is a beginner-level workout because it is simple to perform and does not require any equipment. Mountain climbing is a wonderful aerobic workout alternative to running because it strengthens your core and helps you lose weight, specifically in the lower abs, without aggravating your back discomfort.

<u>Working Out</u>

Start out in a push-up or plank stance with your hands shoulder-width apart and your shoulders directly on top of your wrists. Your back is flat, your glutes are contracted, and your body is straight. This is the starting posture.

Pull your right knee as much as you can towards your chest without allowing your feet to touch the ground. Maintain a tight core and a straight line with your body.

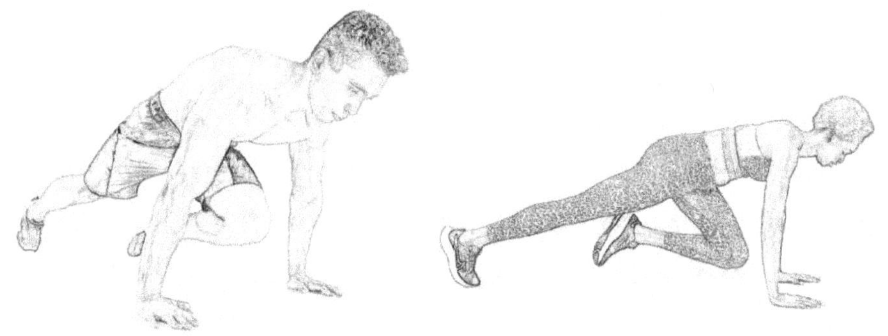

Alternate between bringing your left knee close to your chest and taking the right leg back into the starting position. Maintain a low hip position while switching both knees in and out to generate a "one-two" tempo. With each leg movement, alternate between breathing in and breathing out.

Beginners should practice mountain climbing for 30 seconds. If you find this challenging, you can place your body on an inclined slope by resting both hands on a raised surface, like a chair. This relieves strain on your arms, core, and shoulders. Intermediates should work for 45 to 60 seconds, while advanced students should go for 60 seconds or longer. Once you've mastered the standard variation, seek harder variations to keep yourself challenged.

V-Ups

V-ups are a fantastic core workout that works both your upper and lower abs. You must simultaneously lift your legs and arms off the ground while forming a V shape with just your abdominal muscles. It is comparable to the boat stance for individuals who practice yoga. Imagine this as a single exercise that combines a sit-up and a lying leg raise. The V-Up is a complex exercise that simultaneously engages the muscles in your lower body and core. The rectus abdominis and obliques are the main muscles targeted. The hip flexors, adductors, and quadriceps are the secondary muscles that are engaged.

This workout will greatly improve your ability to walk, run, and lunge in everyday settings. Getting ripped abs while strengthening your hip flexors is like killing two birds with one stone. This exercise works well for beginners because all you need is your body to perform it. However, you will be challenged to improve your balance and coordination because you must contract both the rectus abdominis and the entire abdominal wall in order to balance your arms and legs in the air simultaneously.

<u>Working Out</u>

Start by lying on your back with your arms raised above your head. Lift your feet approximately 6 inches off the ground while keeping them close together and pointed. Engage your core muscles. This is the starting posture.

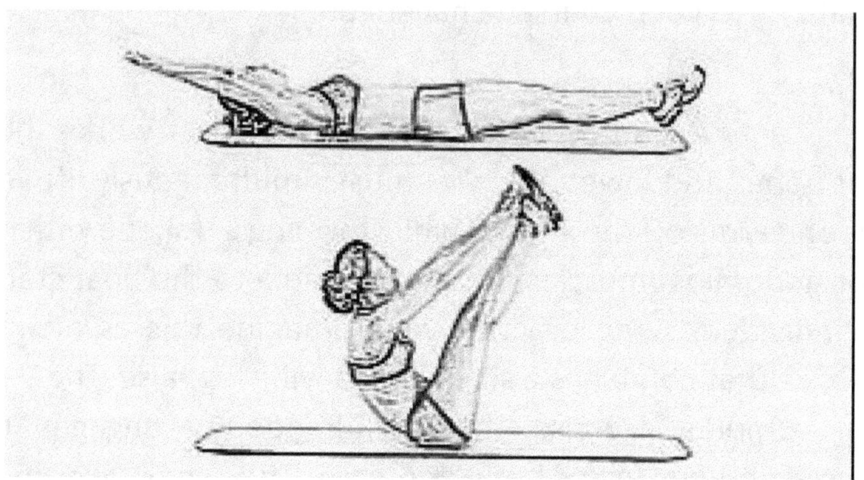

Exhale while lifting your legs and torso at the same time to form a V-shape. Extend your arms so they almost touch your legs. Keep your core engaged and maintain a straight body with your legs and arms.

With your arms aloft and your legs outstretched, inhale as you slowly lower your body to the starting posture. Keep your feet around 6 inches above the ground and slow down your return using your core strength. One rep is completed.

V-ups are fantastic because they will set your abs ablaze. You'll have to rely on your core strength to lift your torso and legs so that they are close to each other. Your upper and lower abs will receive intense treatment throughout this exercise, giving you a well-chiseled core. Once you have mastered the standard version, seek other variations to keep your body challenged.

Plank/Planche

The plank serves as an isometric core workout that requires you to keep your body in an upright position. This exercise works a variety of muscle groups simultaneously, strengthening your core while also exercising your shoulders, glutes, and arms. The reason this exercise is called 'Plank' is because, when performed properly, your body will straighten and remain firm just like a plank of wood.

According to research, a firm core is crucial for transmitting power over the limbs and preventing spinal disturbances during physical exercise. A stronger core can also improve trunk stability and athletic performance while significantly reducing the risk of lower-back issues. When you hold a plank, your body is balanced on your toes and forearms; the bulk of the work in a plank is performed by your core muscles. The obliques and abdominals are the main muscles used. The anterior deltoids, trapezius, serratus anterior, rhomboids, and glutes are the secondary muscles that are engaged.

The plank is a beginner-level exercise that is quick to perform and a wonderful addition to your training regimen because it doesn't call for any special equipment. The plank position is quite simple to take, and for people who find it too simple, there are numerous difficult versions.

<u>Working Out</u>

Elbow Plank: Start out in a plank position, toes and forearms flat on the ground, with shoulders directly on the elbows. Put your palms firmly on the floor or hold a grip. With your head relaxed, look down between your hands.

To keep your body in a straight line, contract your glutes and core. You shouldn't have a high or sagging buttock. The neutral spine posture is shown here. Ensure you maintain a steady breath.

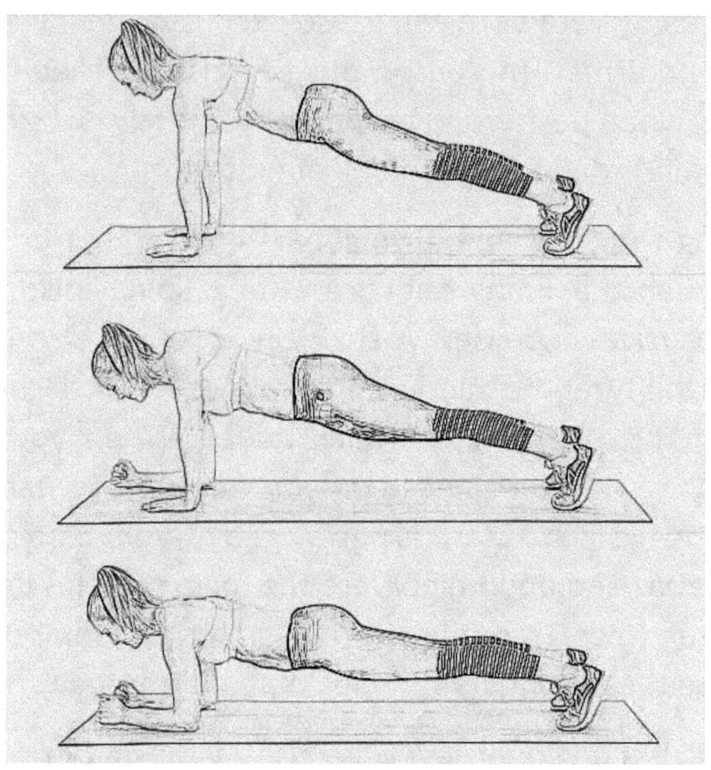

Hold off on the posture for as long as you can stretch. Your duration will get longer when you commit to it more often. 10–120 seconds in 5 sets is recommended.

High Plank: Start in a push-up or plank stance with your arms at shoulder width and your shoulders directly over your wrists. Your feet are straight on the ground.

Your body should be tight, in a straight line from your head to your heels, with your glutes and core engaged. Your hips shouldn't sag, and your back should stay straight and not arched. Maintain a constant breathing rate.

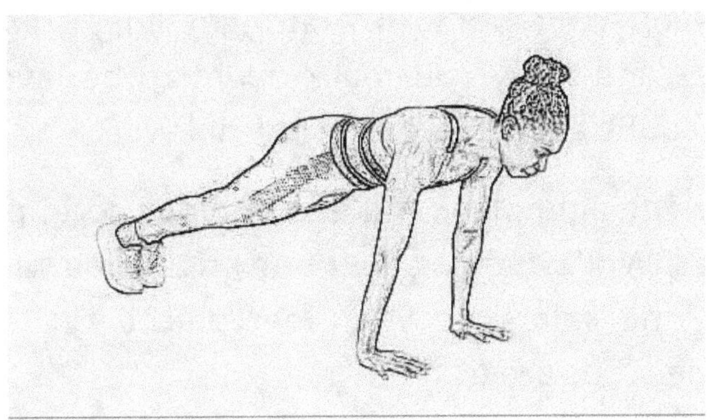

Hold this posture for the longest time possible. 10–120 seconds in 5 sets is recommended.

Common variations of this exercise include:

Knee Plank: The most basic variation of a plank is the knee plank. This exercise is made considerably simpler by having you do a plank on your knees rather than your toes, which takes the strain off your core. Either a high plank or an elbow plank can be used for this exercise. To achieve this, you must:

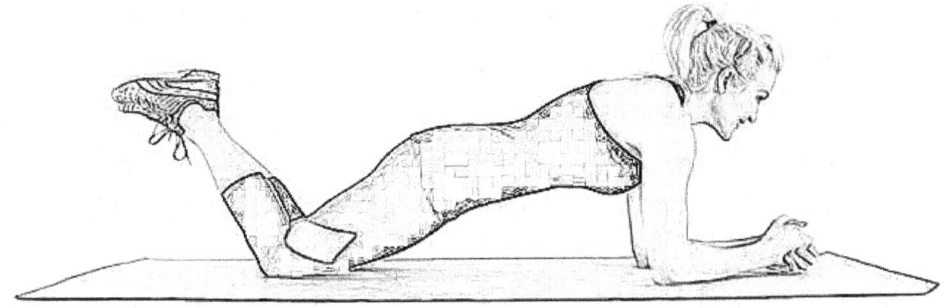

- Set up an elbow or high plank with your hands on the ground, elbows directly beneath your shoulders, and core tightened. Your feet remain in the air as you lower your knees to the ground.

- To keep your body in a straight line, contract your glutes and core. Your back ought to be level and not curved. Be sure to breathe normally.

Side Plank: The side plank focuses on your core, particularly the obliques. While keeping your body rigid, you will rest your weight on one side with your feet placed on top of one another. The steps are as follows:

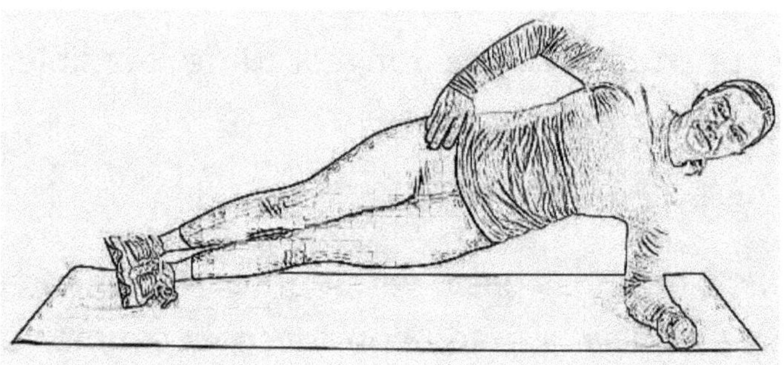

- Lay on your right side, tucking your right elbow beneath your right shoulder and pointing your forearm forward. Make a fist with your hand, with your feet piled on top of one another and your legs straight. Your left hand should be on your waist.
- Make sure your body is tight and in a straight line from head to feet by contracting your glutes, quads, and core. Maintain a steady breathing rhythm with your neck in neutral posture.
- Work on both the left and right sides in one set.

As soon as this variant becomes simple, you can go to a raised side plank.

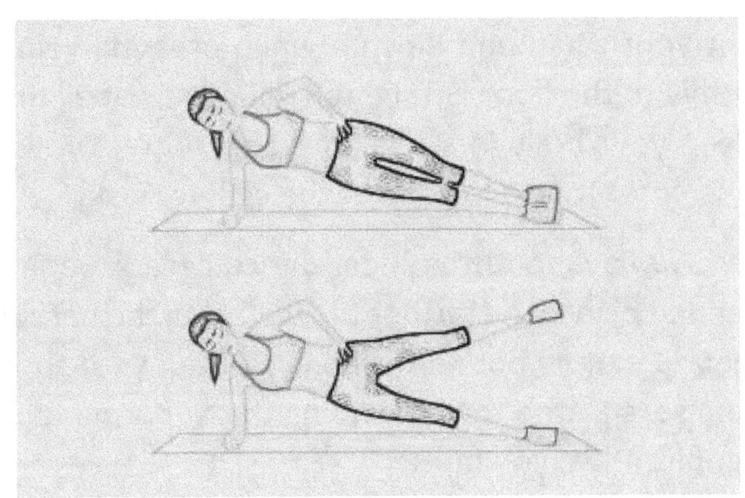

Reverse Plank: Reverse planks work your abdominal muscles, specifically the rectus abdominis, popularly known as the "6 - ack muscle." The glutes are also worked. This workout is appropriate for beginners and would be an excellent bonus to your core program. It is strongly advised that you incorporate this into your circuit. To accomplish this, you must:

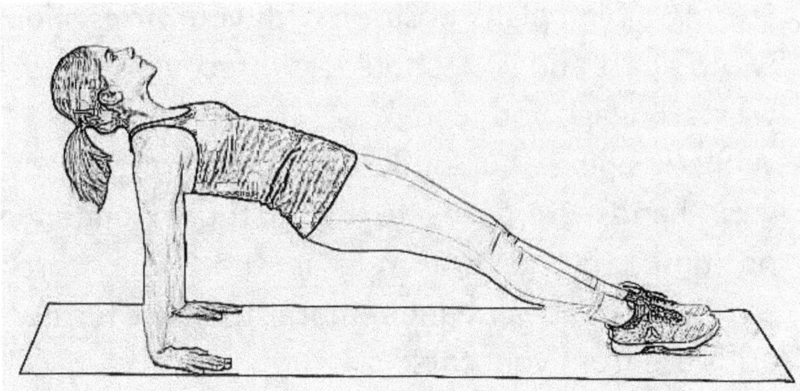

- Start by taking a floor-sitting position and extending your legs in front of you. Put your palms shoulder-width apart on the ground with your fingers pointing in the direction of your feet.

- Lift your torso and hips up while pressing your palms firmly to the floor. Straighten your arms at all times. To keep your body in a straight line, contract your glutes and core. Take a look up at the ceiling or sky.

Extended Plank: One of the most difficult plank variations is the extended plank. The farther the distance, the harder it will be for you to extend both arms up in front of your shoulders. This exercise is a step towards doing the Superman push-up. To accomplish this, you must:

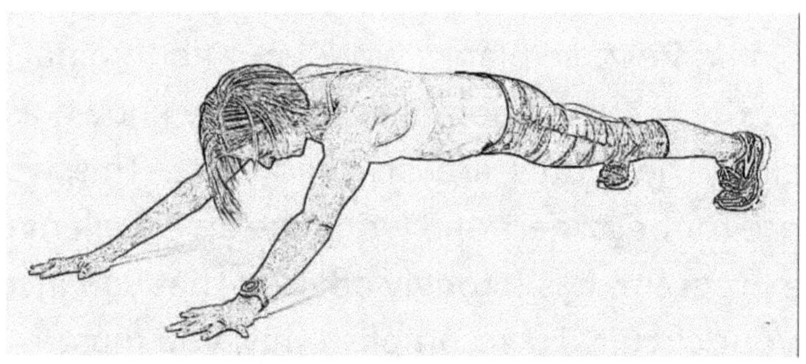

- Start in a high plank position with your arms shoulder-width apart and your shoulders directly on top of your wrists. Engage your core.
- While keeping your body tight and straight, advance your hands 2-4 steps to be in the extended plank position. The general rule is that your core and shoulders will be put under more stress the farther your arms are from your torso.
- To enhance the intensity, you should progressively advance your hands.

Wide-Leg Plank: The wide-leg plank is a simple variant that can strengthen your balance and stability while toning your core. The exercises are easier because of the wide-legged stance, but the muscles of the lower body are still worked.

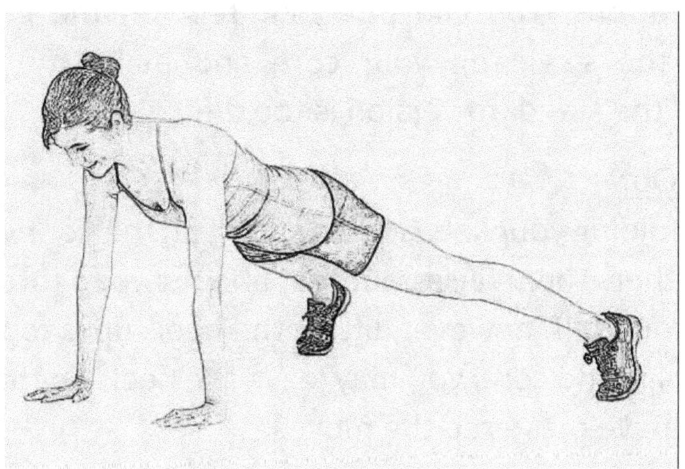

- Start off in a plank position with your arms shoulder width apart, your shoulders directly on the top of your wrists, and your feet apart.
- To keep your body in a straight line, engage your core, hamstrings, glutes, and hip flexors.
- To enhance the intensity, you should progressively advance your hands.

Russian Twists

The Russian Twist is an excellent workout for strengthening your entire core, especially the obliques. It also works your shoulders and hips. In this workout, you will sit up straight with both feet off the floor while rotating your torso from side to side. This rotational movement is frequently used in sports, making it a well-liked exercise for athletes. The Russian twist is believed to have been created by the former Soviet Union as a drill exercise for Russian soldiers during the Cold War.

The Russian Twist is a great exercise for beginners because it's easy to complete and you'll feel the burn in your abs after a few repetitions. You can put your feet on the ground to mitigate the strain on your core and make the exercise simpler if the standard version is too difficult.

<u>Working Out</u>

Begin by folding your knees while sitting on the floor with your feet together. Then, raise your feet about two to three inches off the ground. If, however, lifting the heels up is too difficult for your hips and core, you may leave the heels on the ground until you have mastered the move.

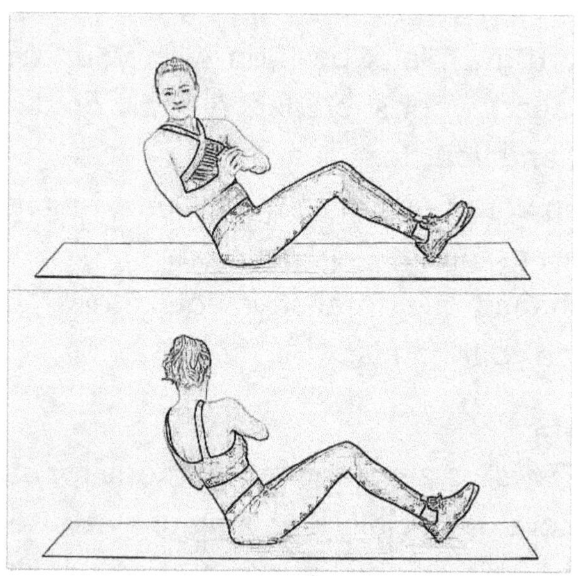

Maintain a strong core and lengthen and straighten your spine at an angle of 45 degrees, forming a V with your thighs and torso. Starting the Russian Twist without your back rounding forward will protect your spine from harm. Your fingers should be intertwined or flat in the middle of your chest.

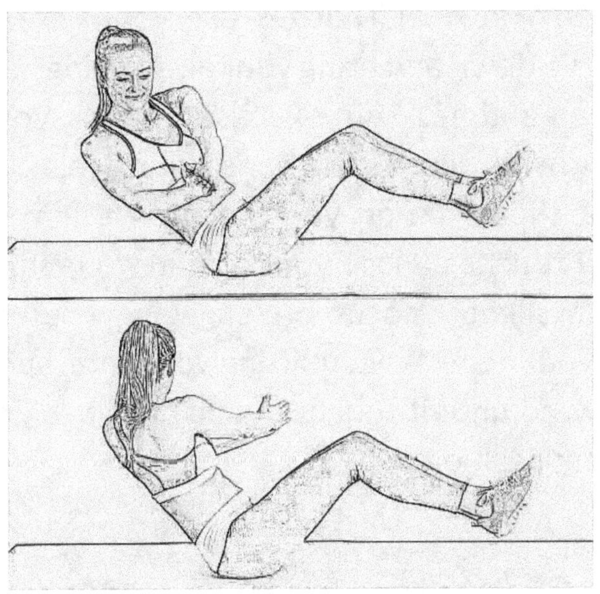

Turn your torso to the left while rotating from your core. Only twist your torso; do not twist your head! Your shoulder should rotate as much in each direction as is feasible with each twist. Maintain a neutral position for your neck. Exhale each time you turn, then breathe back in each time you come back to the starting point. Proper breathing can reduce stress and muscular tension, soothe your nerves, improve your focus, and, most significantly, lessen fatigue and increase stamina.

Perform this action for four sets of 30–60 seconds each.

Variations

This Russian Twist variation will help you tone your obliques while keeping your workouts enjoyable and varied. You can develop new motivation by adding variations to it and switching up your exercises in your program, which will eventually lead to more improvement.

Heel Touches: The Heel Touches use your core muscles to tense as you lie down and bring your alternating hands to your heels, one at a time. This exercise targets your abs and obliques. With your knees bent and your heels close to your bottom, you should lie on your back on a flat surface and execute heel touches. Place your arm at your side with your shoulders up slightly; focus on engaging your abdominals rather than your neck. Next, utilizing your core, spin your right hand downward until it touches your right heel, then return to the starting position.

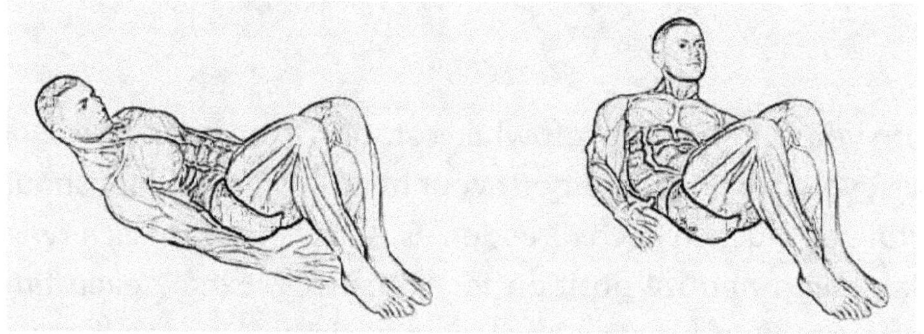

Repeat the identical action on the left side and switch sides until your desired number of repetitions have been completed.

Squat Exercises

Without a powerful and well-developed lower body, no physique is complete. Lower-body workouts should be a regular aspect of your fitness regimen. The amazing thing about these workouts is that you can work your glutes, calves, and thighs without any special equipment. Your lower body has some of the most powerful muscles. The hips, buttocks, and legs must all be strong enough to execute daily duties comfortably. Each task, such as walking, climbing, and sitting, is made easier by improving agility and balance by building and maintaining the strength of these muscles.

Furthermore, lower-body calisthenics workouts improve muscle balance and symmetry. Focusing only on upper body training can result in muscular imbalances that not only seem unusual but also increase the chance of injury, such as inner knee pain. Lower-body exercises help calisthenics athletes develop full-body control and coordination. Lower body movements necessitate precise motor skills and body awareness, which contribute to enhanced balance and coordination. These qualities are required for perfecting advanced calisthenic workouts that require fluid transitions and intricate movements.

Bodyweight Squat
The bodyweight squat is a basic calisthenics exercise that improves leg muscle definition and strength. It is a beginner-level exercise because it is simple to perform and can be done anywhere. It's a highly functional action that works all of the major muscles in the legs. The quadriceps, glutes, and hamstrings are the key muscles targeted. The abdominals, calves, lower back, and hip flexors are secondary muscles.

<u>Working Out</u>

Stand shoulder-width apart with your feet shoulder-width apart, your back straight, your chest out, and your shoulders down. You should have your toes pointed slightly outward. Keep your core engaged.

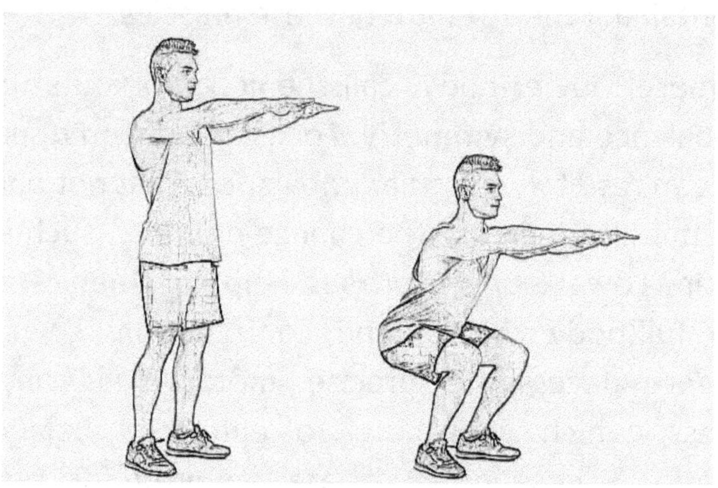

Inhale and start the action by first hinging at the hips, then bending the knees. Continue to descend until your thighs are parallel to the ground; if your ankle flexibility allows you to descend farther, do so. Ensure that your knee is pointed in the same direction as your big toe, and bring both arms out in front of you to balance. In this position, your back should be straight and long. If your back is rounded, drop as much as you can while keeping your back straight.

Exhale and press your heels together to straighten your legs, with your hips and torso rising at the same time. Maintain a flat back by engaging your core all through this action.

Repeat this movement as many times as you want.

<u>Variations</u>

Bodyweight Jump Squats: This version is a step up from bodyweight squats. It is an intermediate-level workout that is excellent for developing explosive power. Additionally, due to the jump, it burns calories more quickly than Bodyweight Squats. It will allow you to take off and move faster, which is something that athletes in sports like football and tennis aspire for. To burst off the ground, press both feet down and leap as high as you can, landing securely with your toes touching the ground first.

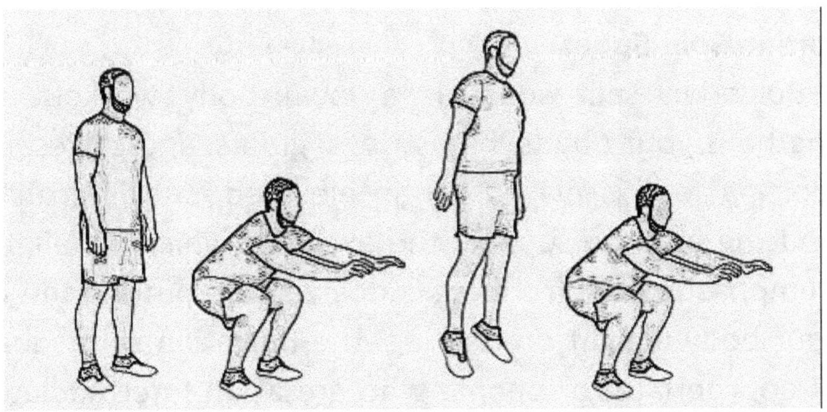

Sumo Squats: Sumo Squats are an entry-level exercise that employs the same muscles used in the Bodyweight Squat. The only difference is that your feet are now wider apart and more turned outward, causing your hips to externally spin. This increases the focus on your abductors and inner thighs.

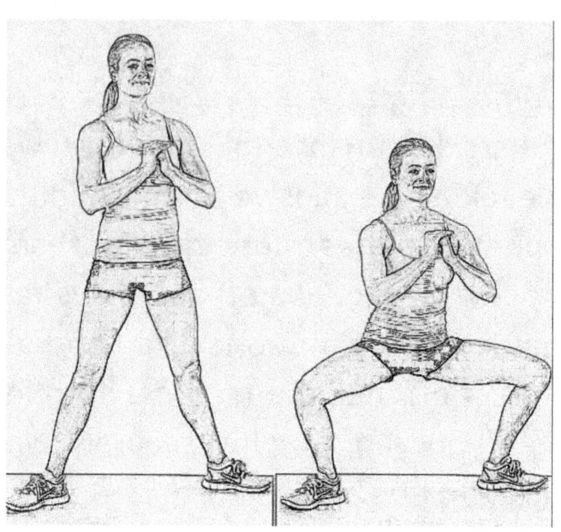

Bulgarian Split Squat

The Bulgarian split squat is a lower-body workout that strengthens your quads, hamstrings, glutes, and calves. The supporting foot is placed on an elevated, sturdy structure behind the body to support the exercise, which is unilateral and emphasizes the front leg. Since you are putting the bulk of your body weight on one leg, the Bulgarian split squat is most appropriate for people who are at an intermediate or higher level. To maintain proper form, better coordination and balance across the entire body are needed.

<u>Working Out</u>

Locate a raised surface, such as a bench, chair, or other piece of furniture, where you can put your back foot down. During this workout, your front leg functions as the working leg, and your back leg will be employed as a support for balance. You have the option of placing your back foot flat or on the toes.

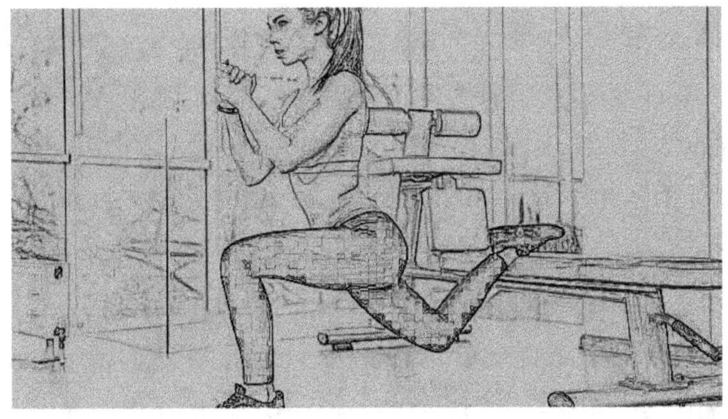

You should start by bending your front knee until it is behind your toes in the sweet spot when your body is straight.

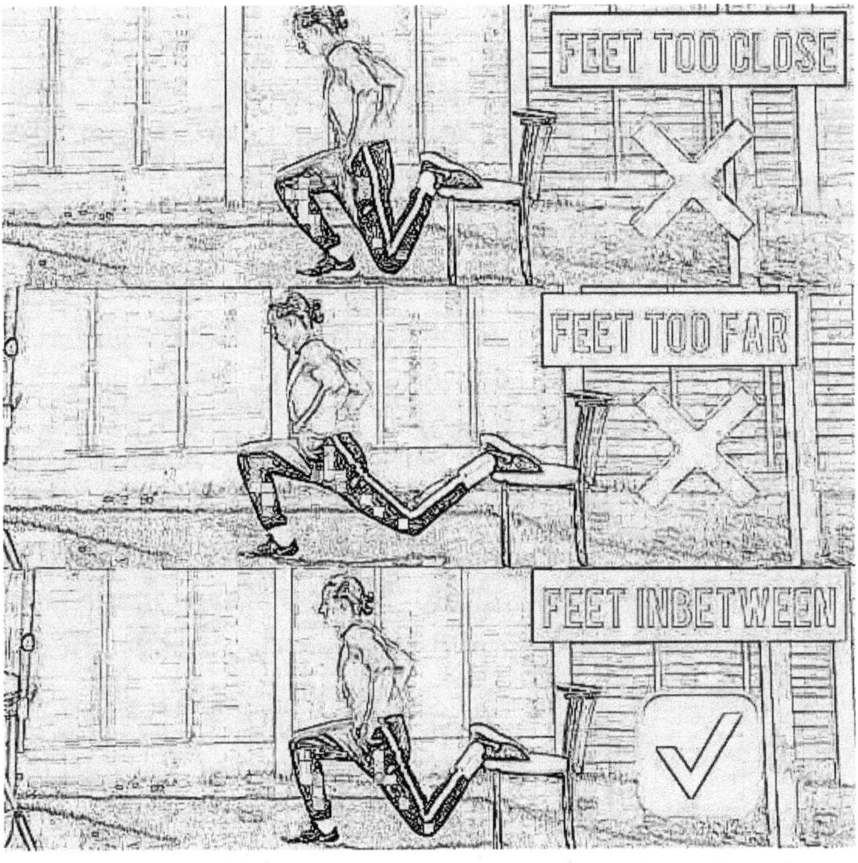

FEET TOO CLOSE

FEET TOO FAR

FEET INBETWEEN

Maintain a tight core at all times while keeping your hips forward and square. This will guarantee that you keep your form correct throughout the movement. Inhale and slowly lower yourself until your front thighs are parallel to the ground. Have a straight back, and your chest should be kept up. Aim to keep your knees from crossing your toes. To maintain balance, you can keep your arms at your sides or in front of you. It is very important that your back knee never touches the ground; therefore, take control of that eccentric period by transitioning down slowly and steadily.

Lunges
One of the best workouts for building strength and endurance in your lower body is the lunge. Lunges are something you probably already know how to do because they are practical and natural; you probably do them every day without even realizing it. For instance, when you stoop to tie your shoelaces or put on your shoes, The quadriceps, glutes, and hamstrings are the main muscles used in lunges. The abdominal and calf muscles are the supporting muscles.

<u>Working Out</u>
Put your left foot back and your right foot forward to form a split stance. Your hips should be squared up and facing forward, and your feet should be roughly three to four feet apart.

By bending your knees at a 90-degree angle, you can lower your body while maintaining a straight upper body, strong abs, and a straight torso. Make sure your left knee is behind the right toe and that your left thigh is parallel to the floor.

The hind leg's knee should be just off the floor. Keep the sole of your front foot firmly planted.

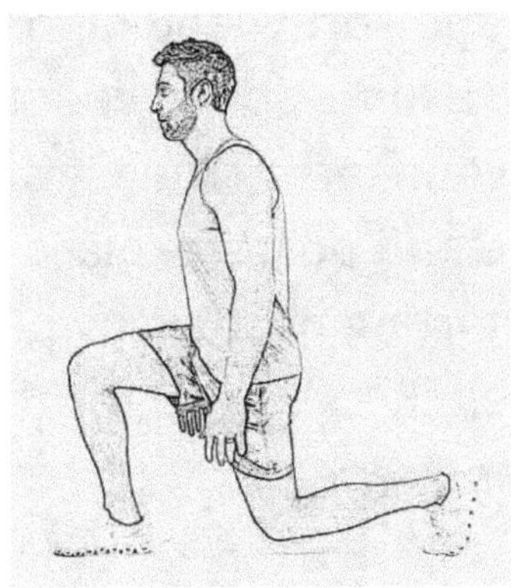

After completing the predetermined number of repetitions, switch to the left leg and perform the same number of repetitions.

<u>Variations</u>

Side/Lateral Lunges: Start by taking a tall stance with your feet hip-width apart. Take a long stride (about three to four feet) to the right. Pushing your hips back, bend your right knee. Throughout this motion, be sure that both feet are planted firmly on the ground. To get back to your starting position, push off using the left leg. Put this into action for the specified number of reps. Switch legs and repeat.

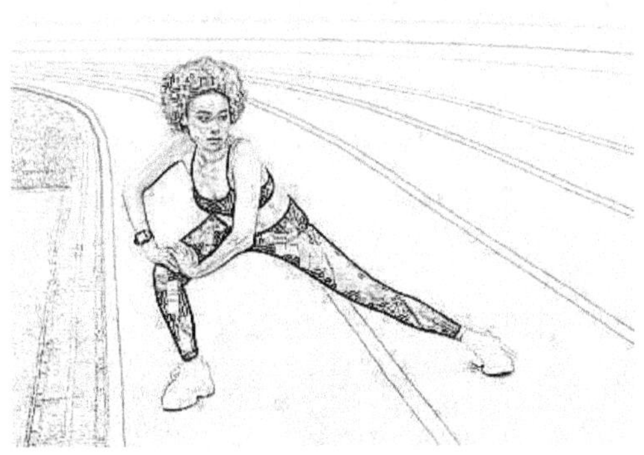

Reverse Lunges: Start by taking a tall stance with your feet hip-width apart. Take a step back with the right foot, keeping your heel off the ground and softly landing onto your right foot's ball. As you drop into a lunge, bend your knees at about a 90-degree angle. Keep your torso straight and your core active. To keep your balance and posture, place both hands on your hips. Return to the starting posture by pushing with the heel of the left foot as well. Repeat this for the specified number of reps. Switch legs and repeat.

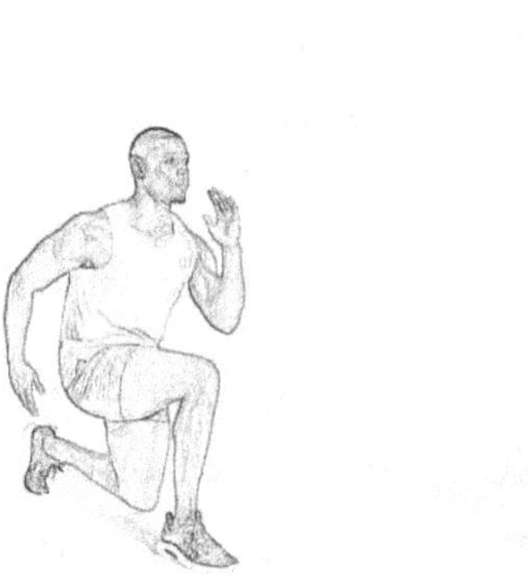

Curtsey Lunges: Start by taking a tall stance with your feet hip-width apart. Move your right foot counterclockwise to the left, drawing a semicircle, until it passes behind your left foot. To aid in finding balance, place both hands on your hips or clasp them in front of your chest. Continue to tuck your right toe. Lunge down until your knees are about 90 degrees down. Your right knee is meant to be about an inch or two off the ground. Slowly make your way back to the starting standing curtsey position. Repeat this for the specified number of times. Switch legs and repeat in the same rep and set.

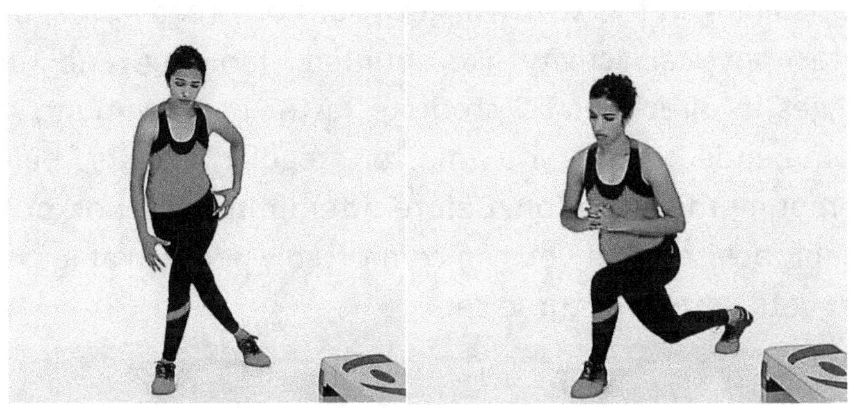

Due to the fact that lunges are unilateral movements, just one side of your body is worked out at a time. As you lunge during this exercise, your body is thrown off balance, which forces your core and abdominal muscles to be active. A strong core will help you improve your balance and posture and reduce back pain. Your balance will gradually improve the more lunges you do and the more variations you utilize. Lunges help your body's ability to balance by training your proprioceptive nerves to respond to position changes more quickly.

This exercise will help you get a tighter butt and sculpt it to improve its overall appearance. People frequently perform squats to achieve the desired butt-shaping effects; nevertheless, lunges are just as beneficial, if not more so, because they improve balance and coordination.

Pistol Squats
The pistol squat is a challenging lower-body workout that targets one leg at a time. Being on one leg while performing a

full squat will help you develop unilateral strength. Pistol squats put your balance, strength, and coordination to the test. Training in this way will get your body ready for sports-related physical activity like sprinting, jumping, and rapid changes in direction. To promote faster improvement, it is recommended that you master regular squats before attempting this variation. Before attempting this workout, it is highly advised that you can comfortably perform at least 15 air squats for two or three sets.

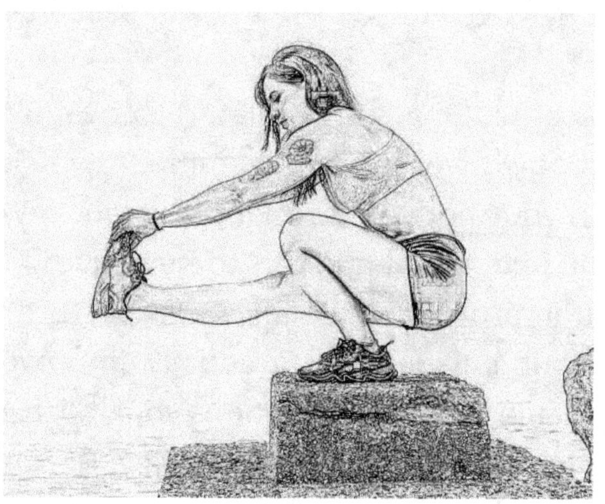

<u>Working Out</u>

Before engaging in any squatting workout, it's crucial to stretch out your calves and ankles and relieve any stiffness or tightness. Stretching both before and after exercising will increase your strength and flexibility, which will help you feel less pain and have a wider range of motion.

Progression to the Pistol Squat:

You can start using these three efficient pistol squat progressions right away to build the power, balance, and coordination needed for the pistol squat. Since these progressions are graded from simple to hard, you can decide which ones are appropriate for your present level of fitness and incorporate them into your training program accordingly. For best results, do this routine a minimum of twice a week.

<u>Deep Squat:</u> A deep squat is one in which your hips are lowered below the level of your knees. The idea is to be able to attach your glutes to your calves. Your calves and ankles will become more mobile as a result of this exercise, increasing your pistol squat range of motion. Holding onto a solid object in front of you will provide support as you practice deep squats. The steps are as follows:

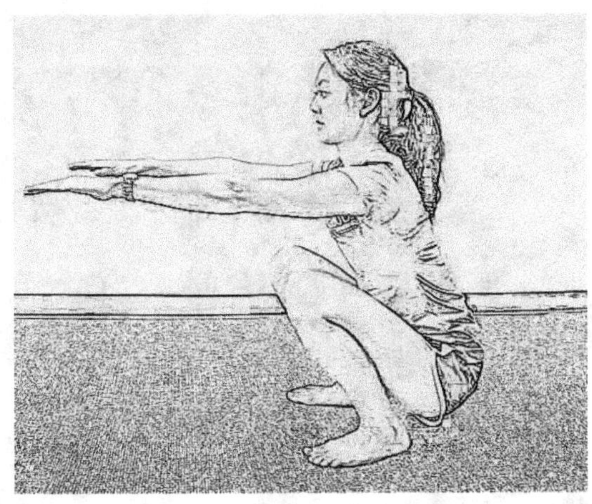

- o Standing tall and with your feet slightly pointing outside, space them shoulder-width apart. This is the starting posture.
- o Inhale and bend your knees and hips as if you were sitting on a chair. Maintain a straight torso by engaging

your core. Your heels should stay flat on the floor while you squat until your hips are at knee level. If you find this challenging, you can hold onto the chair in front of you.

- o Exhale as you push down your heels to go back to where you were. Squeeze your glutes while standing back on top.
- o Rep this movement 5–12 times for 4 sets.

<u>Pistol Box Squat</u>: Due to the pistol box squat's restricted range of motion, the targeted muscles will gain strength and stamina. As you gain strength, lower the box's height to make the challenge harder. The steps are as follows:

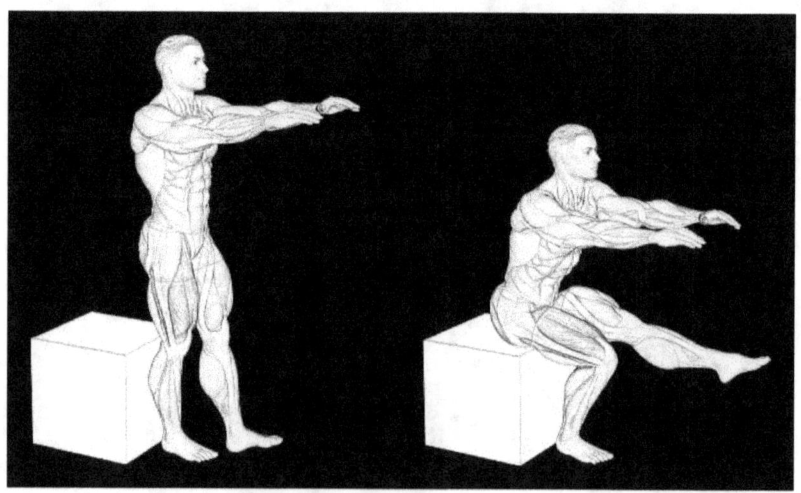

- o Stand erect in front of an elevated item, like a chair or a plyometric box, with your feet hip-width apart.
- o Inhale while bringing your hips back and bending your right knee. Maintain a firm core. Your buttocks should touch the box as you descend. To balance yourself, extend your left leg and arms in front of you.

o Exhale out as you raise yourself back up to upright posture by pushing through your heel. Squeeze your quads and glutes while standing back up.
o Perform 5–12 reps on each leg for four sets.

Assisted Pistol Squat: With the assistance of hanging on an item such as gymnastic rings, the TRX, a rail, or a chair, this exercise is excellent for developing the entire range of motion needed for the pistol squat. This will help you with balance as well as support some of your body's weight by removing the load from your leg, allowing you to lift less. To accomplish this, you must:

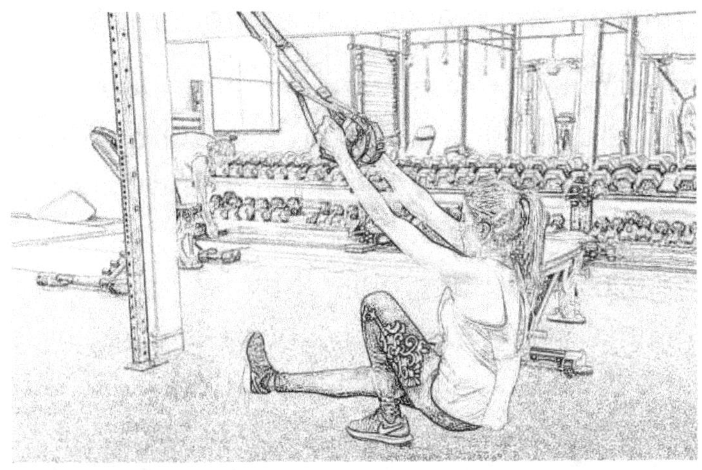

o Place both feet hip-width apart and stand tall. Grab a strong object from your side, like a table, a rail, or a bar. For additional assistance, try gymnastics rings or the TRX.
o Squat down on the right leg while holding the object in both hands. Maintain a straight torso by engaging your

core. To balance yourself, extend your left leg in front of you. Inhale while performing this move.

- o As you climb to standing, exhale and plant your heel firmly on the ground. Instead of pulling up with your arms, use your legs to push up.
- o Perform 5 to 12 repetitions on a single leg for 4 sets.

Executing a Pistol Squat:

After you've completed the previous three progressions, you can move on to the full pistol squat, which involves a single-leg full squat. The objective is to squat down until your glute contacts your calf. Here are the required steps:

- o The toes of your right leg should be pointed forward when you stand tall. To activate your quadriceps, raise the opposite leg off the ground and extend it out in front of you a little.
- o Inhale as you drop yourself as far as you can on the standing leg, keeping your body straight by engaging your core. To counterbalance, extend your left leg and both hands forward.
- o Exhale as you push through the heel of your right leg to return to the initial standing posture
- o Squeeze your glutes and quadriceps while standing back up.
- o Perform 3–10 repetitions on a single leg for 4 sets.

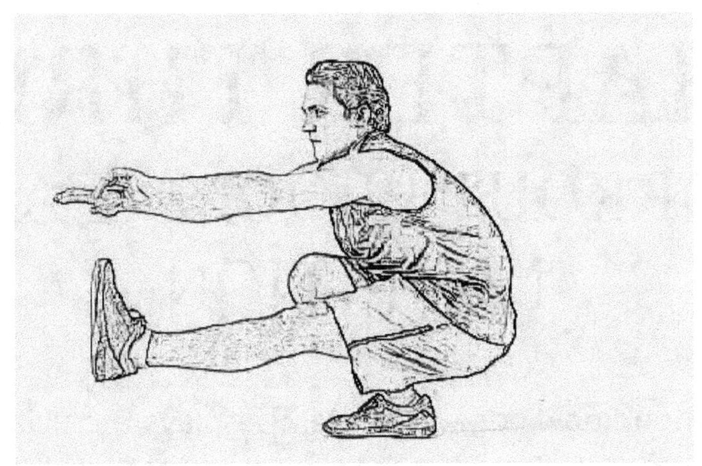

Pistol squats improve leg tension because your full body weight is carried on a single leg. Your muscles may experience additional stress as a result of this isolated exercise, which could result in increased strength and muscle development. When you build your weak side through unilateral exercise, you will definitely see improvements in your standard bilateral squats, which work both legs at the same time.

CHAPTER THREE
WORKOUT PROGRAM AND NUTRITION

It's common knowledge that exercise plays a crucial role in maintaining both your physical and mental well-being. It encompasses everything, from managing your weight to preserving muscle mass, enabling you to perform daily tasks effortlessly. Moreover, it assists in indulging in occasional treats without guilt. From the outset, it's imperative to understand that you cannot out-train a poor diet, nor can exercise alone eliminate excess body fat. This underscores the paramount importance of establishing a consistent routine, akin to the adage that "abs are made in the kitchen."

For beginners embarking on their fitness journey, the emphasis should not be on leaping from zero to a hundred right away. Instead, focus on finding equilibrium and constructing a solid foundation. It's advisable to keep your workouts within the 60-minute mark or less. Oftentimes, what doesn't happen in the first hour of your workout will not happen in the second.

Full Body vs Split Training

Split training, also known as bro split, is usually the default type of training used by bodybuilders. With a very basic split training routine, you will be setting up your workout in a way where you will be focusing only on one muscle or one muscle group per day.

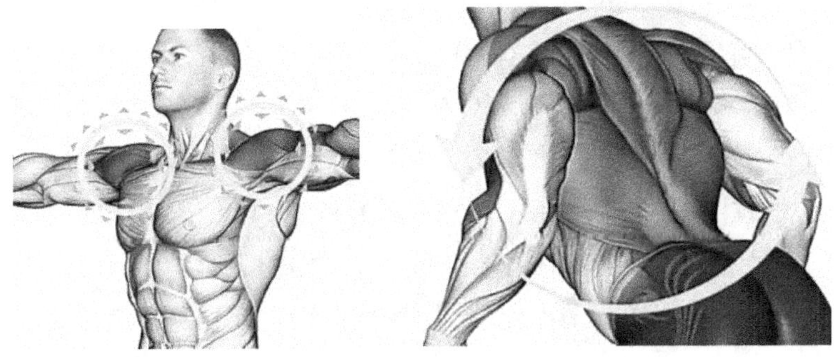

So, a typical basic split training routine might look like this:

- Monday – Chest Day
- Tuesday – Back Day
- Wednesday – Leg Day
- Thursday – Shoulders and Abs
- Friday – Biceps and Triceps
- Saturday – Off Day (Rest)
- Sunday – Off Day (Rest)

Then you start the routine again the following week by going back to the chest.

On the other hand, with full-body training, it is obvious you are working your entire body in every single section. That means, unlike bro split training, you are working your chest, arms, back, and abs all in one day. Usually, a typical full-body training routine will see you working out three times a week with one day off in between each section. So, Monday – Wednesday – Friday will be a full body workout. And then the rest of the week can be used as off.

Now, if you want to build muscle and increase lean body mass, you need to focus on increasing the volume of your workout. And volume is measured by four factors: intensity, frequency, sets, and reps. Increasing any of these four factors will help you build more muscle. Now, you may start to notice the advantage that a full-body workout provides over a basic split training routine. They require fewer days for exercise, and you will be targeting all the muscles in your body three times a week, every week, as opposed to split training, where you will only be targeting each muscle once a week.

That means that you will be increasing that frequency factor much higher with full body training, and even if you do spend an entire workout section beating up your chest in a split training routine, it shouldn't take longer than a maximum of three to four days for your chest to recover, which means you will miss out on potential muscle gains since you will be waiting seven days to work your chest again instead of four days.

So, to make up for this lack of frequency, other split training routines have grown in popularity, such as:

- Push-pull routines
- Opposing body part routines
- Upper and lower routines

A push-pull routine focuses on grouping your push muscles (i.e., chest, shoulders, and triceps) separately from your pull muscles (i.e., back and biceps). A typical routine might look something like this:

- Day 1 – Chest, Shoulders and Triceps
- Day 2 – Legs and Abs
- Day 3 – Back and Biceps
- Day 4 – Rest

Then repeat, which would allow you to hit each muscle group twice a week.

With an opposing body part routine, you would group two opposing muscle groups, like your chest and back, into one workout, and each time you performed a set for your chest, you would immediately perform another set with no break for your back. By doing this, you would be able to work heavily on each muscle since each exercise works primarily different muscles, and you could save time by pairing the two sets together. A sample routine will be:

- Day 1 – Chest and Back
- Day 2 – Hamstring and Quad Movement
- Day 3 – Shoulders, Biceps, and Triceps
- Day 4 – Rest

This would again allow you to work each muscle twice a week.

The upper and lower routine simply involves working your entire upper body one day and your entire lower body the next day. A typical routine will be:

- Monday – Upper Body
- Tuesday – Lower Body
- Wednesday – Rest
- Thursday – Upper Body
- Friday – Lower Body
- Weekend – Off (Rest and Recover)

Now, with both of these programs in mind, here are some vital points to consider in order to make a decision:

- ❖ If you are a total beginner, you will be better off solidifying your form and execution with a full- body program that incorporates key compound exercises in order to develop a very strong foundation.
- ❖ If you are too busy to have a 5- to 6-day routine in a week, you will probably benefit more from a full-body routine.
- ❖ If you have been training for some time and have noticed any lagging muscle groups that you would like to improve, i.e calves, chest, etc. If you want to isolate these muscles, work on catching them up to speed with the rest of your body. You will probably be better off with split training.
- ❖ If you are someone who is ready to work the same muscle groups every other day because your body recovers quickly, then full-body training could be a good fit.
- ❖ If you are always sore for 3–4 days at a time, you may want to give your muscles more time to recover in between sessions with split training.

❖ If your goal is to build a perfectly proportional physique such that the size of your calves matches the size of your biceps, you will be better off with split training. On the other hand, if you just want to burn some fat, increase your conditioning, or are a busy person who just wants to stay in shape and be healthy without spending a ton of time working out, a full-body routine will be suitable.

Tips for Effective Workout Program

Identify Specific Goal: It may sound like basic advice, but it's a crucial point that often gets overlooked. Defining your specific end goal is essential. Are you aiming to increase your strength, build muscle, lose fat, or achieve a combination of these objectives? While most goals share common foundations like proper nutrition, resistance training, and sufficient sleep, each goal has distinct requirements.

For instance, building muscle necessitates progressive overload in terms of volume and exertion rather than solely focusing on intensity. Fat loss places significant emphasis on nutrition, with exercise following a more flexible progression approach. Strength gains often rely on periodization strategies involving peaks and tapers to optimize your fitness capacity at specific points in your training cycle. Understanding the unique demands of your goal is fundamental to tailoring an effective fitness and nutrition plan.

Adopt a Proven Program First: For beginners, it can be overwhelming to create numerous workout programs with limited knowledge in the field. Watching countless internet videos may not be as helpful as gaining practical experience. It's valuable to learn from those who have already put in the legwork, both literally and figuratively, by following established and proven fitness programs. Doing so not only provides insight into program structure but, more importantly, delivers tangible results.

Once you've accumulated experience and understanding, you can then begin to tailor a program to your specific needs based on your progress and goals. Starting with established programs and gradually customizing them as you become more experienced is a prudent approach to long-term fitness success.

Balance Fitness and Fatigue: Frequently, individuals assume that the solution to plateaus or a lack of results is simply to keep adding more to their workouts. However, the issue may not be that they are not doing enough; it might be that they are pushing themselves too hard, leading to excessive fatigue. This concept aligns with the fatigue-fitness model, which proposes that as fitness improves through training, so does the accumulation of fatigue. Without adequate recovery to manage this fatigue, performance can start to decline, even as fitness adaptations continue to progress. Balancing training intensity with proper recovery becomes crucial to maximizing performance gains over time.

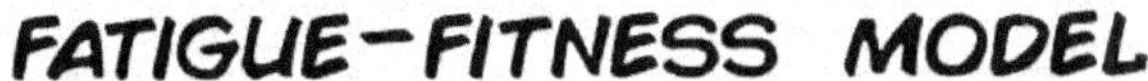

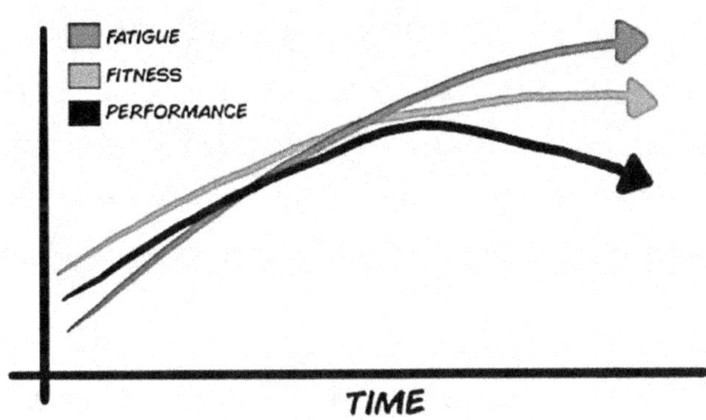

Fatigue is primarily influenced by a high volume of work, so if your training program includes frequent high-volume days, it's advisable to incorporate more recovery days into your schedule. At times, intentionally accumulating fatigue can be a strategic choice, as rebounding from long-term fatigue can position you to perform at your peak within a specific timeframe, a phenomenon known as the overreaching effect.

To maintain a healthy balance between fitness and fatigue, it's crucial to program in periods of deloading and tapering, where work capacity is significantly reduced to allow for adequate recovery. This is typically followed by a peak phase, during which your performance can shine.

Regardless of your training goals, finding the right equilibrium between building fitness and managing fatigue is essential, especially when aiming for optimal performance outcomes.

Measure Reps in Reserve: Choosing the right number of reps can be a bit confusing. Do a few reps, and you won't fully stimulate muscle fibers, thus limiting muscular adaptation. Do too many, especially going to failure, and you might accumulate too much fatigue early on. Which will negatively impact performance or subsequent sets and workouts. The answer, then, is to find a sweet spot where you are training with a lot of effort without accumulating unnecessary fatigue. This is probably the best gauge through something called Reps in Reserve.

Reps in reserve (RIR) represent the number of repetitions you believe you could have performed before reaching failure if you had pushed a given set to its limits. For instance, if you complete a set of squats with 10 reps but feel you could have managed 13 before hitting failure, you would say you had 3 reps in reserve (3 RIR). The ideal number of reps in reserve can vary depending on the specific rep range you are training within.

For lower rep ranges, such as 3-5 reps, fewer RIR, typically around 1-2, may be aimed for. In contrast, higher rep ranges, like 15-20 reps, might target 3–4 RIR. Within typical rep ranges, maintaining 1-2 RIR is often recommended because research suggests that this range maximizes muscle stimulation, negating the need to consistently push to failure. However, if you wish to occasionally train to failure, it's advisable to reserve it for your final set during a workout. Generally, programming your sets with 1-3 RIR is considered a best practice for balanced and effective training.

Diet Plan

Calisthenics routines are undertaken with the primary objectives of enhancing fitness, building strength, and achieving an aesthetically pleasing physique. To attain these goals, it is imperative to ensure that the body receives the necessary nutrients. It's important to recognize that there isn't a one-size-fits-all or superior diet plan, as individual body types, goals, and health considerations such as weight loss, weight gain, high blood pressure, high blood sugar, and allergies vary widely.

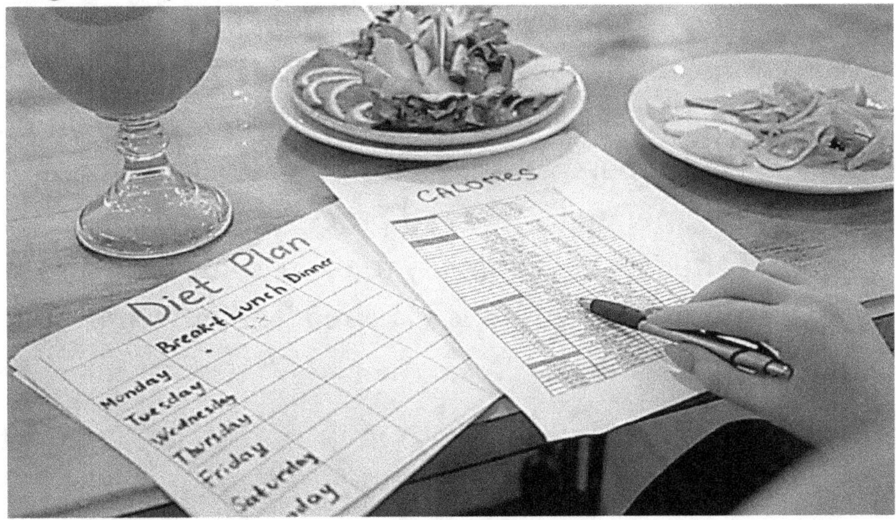

While it may initially appear challenging to pinpoint a diet plan that aligns with your bodyweight fitness aspirations, maintaining a positive mindset is crucial to your success.

Prioritize Protein Intake

Our bodies are made up of proteins, which are especially concentrated in the muscles. Your muscles experience eustress during exercise, causing minute rips in the muscle fibers. These are restored during recuperation by satellite cells, which synthesize protein and make your muscles stronger to prepare for additional exercise.

Eliminate Junk Food

Treating your body as if it were a high-performance sports car means providing it with the premium fuel it needs to maintain its condition and optimize its performance. Just as you would use top-quality fuel for a supercar to keep it running smoothly, our bodies also require the best possible nutrition to achieve their incredible potential.

Steering clear of junk food and highly processed meals that are high in unhealthy fats, sugar, and refined carbohydrates (often referred to as empty carbs) is crucial. These items, including candy bars, sugary treats, cakes, carbonated beverages, sweetened juices, and processed foods, can have detrimental effects on your ability to exercise by sapping your energy, disrupting your metabolism, and leading to unwanted weight gain.

Remember, the fuel you put into your body directly affects how you feel. If you choose to nourish your body with premium-quality fuel, you'll experience the difference, much like a million-dollar Lamborghini hitting the road at its peak performance.

Stay Hydrated

According to the United States Geological Survey, water makes up roughly 60% of your body and plays an important role in bodily function. Every cell needs water to survive, and it first serves as a building block for cells. When you exercise, your body might lose a lot of fluid through breathing and perspiration. Neglecting to replenish this lost fluid can lead to dehydration, which can have adverse effects on both your overall health and your workout performance. Staying adequately hydrated is crucial to ensuring your body functions optimally during exercise and in daily life.

Supplements can Help

Minerals and vitamins play a pivotal role in the proper development and functioning of your body. Although many individuals meet their recommended intake of iron, calcium, and vitamin D through a balanced diet, some may require additional nutritional support, making supplements a viable option.

In the realm of athletic pursuits, supplements have a valuable role to play. They can potentially enhance performance, boost strength, promote lean muscle growth, and alleviate fatigue. It's essential to ensure that you are providing your body with the essential nutrition it needs to maintain optimal health and vigor. However, if you believe you could benefit from additional supplements, here are some worth considering for inclusion in your diet:

Creatine: Enhance training adaptations and exercise capacity using creatine. By allowing people to increase their training volume, these adaptations may promote higher gains in lean mass, muscular strength, and power. Effective dosages range from 2.5 to 5 grams daily.

BCCAs: branched-chain amino acids, or BCCAs This is an essential component in the production of proteins. This promotes muscular growth and lessens post-workout pain in the muscles. A dose of 5g taken at least an hour prior to exercise can be useful.

Multivitamins: Multivitamins are nutritional products that include a wide variety of vitamins and minerals. To stay fit and healthy, our bodies require 13 different vitamins.

Calisthenics Nutrition

Protein	Carbohydrates	Fat
Meat, fish, and poultry (beef, fish, pork, and chicken)	Quinoa, couscous, brown rice, oats, bread, pasta, and lentils	Nuts and seeds
Dairies, i.e yogurt and milk	Fruits and vegetables	Fish, i.e salmon
Beans, i.e lentils, chickpeas	Sweet potatoes and Potatoes	Avocadoes
Nuts	Grains	Olive oil, vegetable oils and olive
Soy and tofu	Cereal	Dark Chocolate

The table provided above offers valuable insights to guide your daily meal planning. It's crucial to ensure that the meals you prepare for yourself are not only nutritious but also enjoyable to eat. A diet lacking in flavor and satisfaction can quickly sap your motivation.

To achieve your dietary goals, it's essential to trust the process and maintain consistency in your meal choices. Monitoring your progress effectively involves weighing yourself at intervals of one to two weeks while also documenting your journey with progress photos. However, it's important to note that daily weigh-ins can have detrimental effects on your mental well-being. These frequent checks can lead to heightened stress and decreased motivation due to natural fluctuations in body weight caused by fluid shifts.

Training Fasted: Training on an "empty tank", as in not eating anything before your workouts, is effective for weight loss but not for strength or performance if you are already very lean.

Pre-Workout Meals: Before working out for the day, you can eat some healthy fats for breakfast or lunch because fats take longer to burn than carbohydrates, and they will keep you energized throughout the day. Also, you can take easily digestible meals, few carbs, and a lot of water. Fruit can also be taken 30 minutes before your first workout.

Consistent calisthenics training will make you fairly shredded by nature, but muscle also grows (hypertrophy) at a slower rate when body fat is extremely low. A body fat percentage of around 9–15% is optimal for calisthenics athletes who want to build muscles. You can consume as much food as you want while following the calisthenics diet, as long as it's nutritious, if you want to see the best results.

CHAPTER FOUR
INJURY PREVENTION AND RECOVERY

Injury management is more than just introducing some injury prevention exercises; it is also how you treat injuries, how you deal with the state of being injured, training in injury, and keeping motivated while being injured.

Relieve Muscle Soreness

The soreness you feel a day or two after a workout is something most people who do calisthenics are familiar with. This feeling, known as Delayed Onset Muscle Soreness (DOMS), is thought to be caused by microscopic tears in your muscle fibers that occur from resistance training or nervous stimulation in general. The cause of DOMS is eccentric contraction, or a muscle becoming longer while under tension. And aside from just being generally comfortable, particularly with leg soreness, too much soreness can also negatively impact your training if it carries over into your next workouts. Studies show that training a muscle while it is still sore can reduce the activation of the desired muscle, reduce the force capacity of the muscle by up to 50%, and negatively interfere with the recovery process.

Therefore, it is vital that you take the necessary steps in order to minimize post-workout soreness and speed up the muscle recovery process. And although two common suggestions are to take ice baths or stretch after a workout, this actually isn't the best advice to take. Although ice baths may slightly help with muscle soreness, they have been shown to hinder muscle growth and strength by interfering with the muscle recovery process. And as for static stretching, multiple studies from the Journal of Sports Medicine have indicated that it actually doesn't help with muscle soreness and may interfere with the recovery process as well. Therefore, both of these wouldn't be the ideal solution for those who want to prioritize muscle growth and strength.

So, aside from the general recommendations of taking adequate protein and getting enough sleep, there are a few extra steps you can take:

Self-Myofascial Release (*Foam Rolling*): This has become increasingly popular in recent years. Aside from its positive effect on improving mobility, it is also an effective way of reducing muscle soreness. And this reduction of muscle soreness seems to enhance the subject's workout performance in their next workouts.

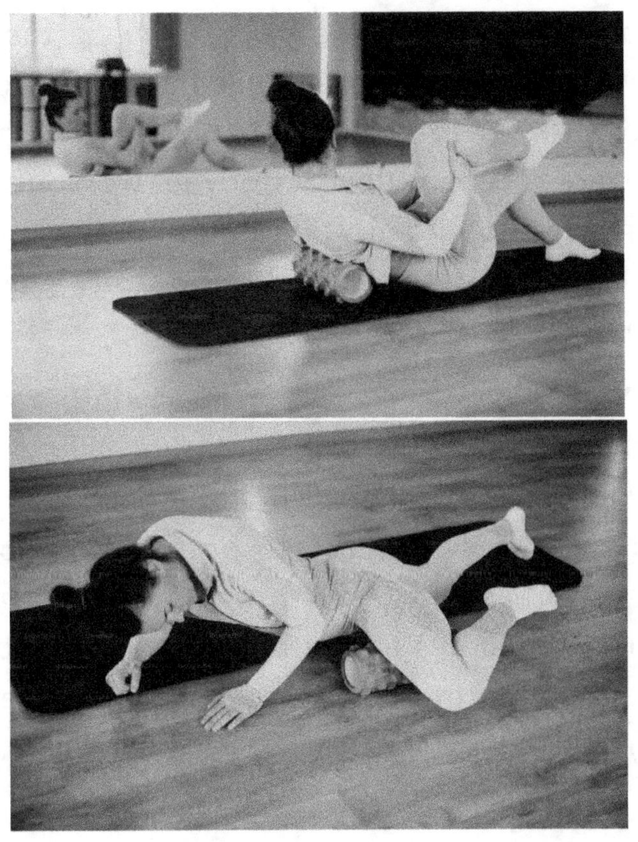

Foam rolling is best done after your workout for around 10 minutes, and stick to the muscles you worked that day, especially the one that tends to experience the most soreness. You can also do the foam rolling a few hours after your workout if that is more convenient for you. Don't go too fast on each muscle, and keep pressure on tight spots until they release.

Active Recovery: Another thing to do to reduce muscle soreness is to incorporate active recovery which includes cooldowns, low- intensity exercise, etc. Some studies have shown that active recovery, whether performed immediately after a workout or within the days following the workout, reduces muscle soreness more than when no active recovery is used. So, in order to implement this, do 5–10 minutes of active recovery or cooling down after your workout, especially for leg workouts. But the most important part when it comes to active recovery is to use a low-intensity exercise that involves the muscles you worked.

Ease into Your Program: Easing your way into a program is the one thing to do that will have the biggest effect on reducing your muscle soreness. If you are a beginner or just starting a new exercise routine, the best thing to do is to take a few weeks to ease into your program. Meaning that you should work at volumes and intensities that are lower than you normally would in order to prevent excessive soreness from occurring.

Elevation: Although these wouldn't work for all muscle parts, elevating the sore area will help reduce the blood flow, reducing the inflammation and swelling. An example could be placing your sore leg on a couch while you lie on the floor.

Painkillers: Whether it is Tylenol, Advil, aspirin, ibuprofen, or something else, the thing you need to keep in mind about painkiller meds is that they relieve the pain and kind of numb you from it so that you are not aware or in touch with which range of motion is further aggravating the affected tissue. So, only take pain meds if you truly cannot bear the pain; otherwise, just avoid the range of motion that hurts, and you will be fine.

Injuring Prevention

To begin with, it's crucial to have a deep understanding of your physical limitations. This involves developing a keen awareness of your body and heeding its signals because, ultimately, no one knows your body better than you do. Overuse injuries often manifest as a result of pushing your body too hard or too fast, and they can also be attributed to repetitive movement patterns.

Injury prevention also entails adequately preparing your muscles, joints, and ligaments for the specific movements you engage in, ensuring that you possess the necessary strength and resilience.

Moreover, our bodies tend to fare better when we introduce variety and avoid repetitive patterns. A simple yet effective strategy for long-term injury prevention is diversifying your grip or altering your movement patterns within your exercise regimen. For instance, when performing exercises like pull-ups on rings or bars, consider alternating between supinated and pronated grips to reduce the risk of overuse injuries.

Treating Injuries

Accelerating the healing process often requires specific measures aimed at improving blood circulation to the affected areas and restoring the strength of the injured tendon or muscle. It's important to note that the healing processes for muscles, ligaments, and joints differ significantly. Therefore, the exercises employed for recovery will largely depend on the nature of the injury.

However, it's essential to understand that, in general, inactivity is the least advisable approach. Staying sedentary can be detrimental to the healing process. Instead, it's crucial to engage in targeted exercises and activities tailored to your injury to promote healing and regain strength.

Training with Injury

A lot of people tend to get stuck in the healing part of an injury and often spend months doing the exercises given to them by their physiotherapist. In some cases, you can actually keep training when you have injuries. And there are quite a few ways this can be approached:

- ✓ Try to adjust the exercises so that they don't hurt, or rather, stay within an acceptable level of pain.
- ✓ There are often ways around injuries, so you should take time to experiment with different variations of the different exercises you do. And learn to know your body and which of these can be performed while injured.
- ✓ If there is no way around the pain, restructure your training and think a bit differently. Find new goals to help you stay motivated while injured. An injury could be a chance for you to catch up on an aspect that you previously neglected, and in some cases, this can actually cause a rejuvenation of your motivation, thereby opening your mind to new aspects of movement.

Setting Up an Injury Gameplan by answering these **Questions:**

1. What can you do to hurry up the healing process?
2. What can you do without the pain being too severe?
3. What other relevant exercises can you do to stay motivated?

CHAPTER FIVE
CALISTHENICS EQUIPMENT

We are all aware that bodyweight exercises, or calisthenics, may be performed without any special equipment. In fact, all you need to perform common calisthenic exercises like pushups, diamond pushups, bodyweight squats, leg lifts, and other exercises is a flat surface, which is easy to obtain nowadays.

However, if you're committed to progressing from a beginner to an elite in this field, it's essential to elevate your training regimen by incorporating some fundamental calisthenics equipment. This equipment not only enables you to target your muscles differently but also enhances the level of challenge while facilitating muscle confusion within your workouts.

Pull-Up Bar

Now, if you want to start doing calisthenics, you absolutely need this piece of equipment. You'll need a pull-up bar whether you're exercising at home or at the office. Pull-ups are the most efficient way to shape your back while also focusing on your core, biceps, and other muscular groups. It is an essential upper-body complex exercise that you cannot perform without a bar over your head. There are many different kinds, and the one that is best for you depends on your housing situation.

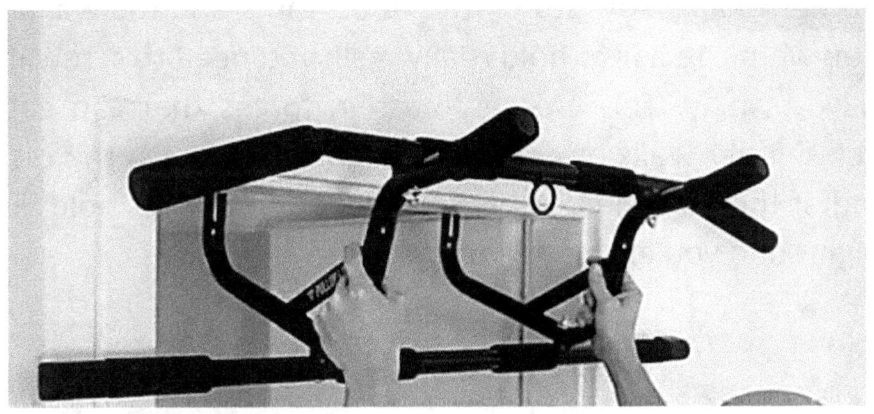

A doorway pull-up bar, like the one in the image above, can be used if you don't have enough room for a free-standing pull-up bar. It's simple to set up and compatible with any door as long as it has a sturdy frame surrounding it. This one doesn't need screws and can support as much as 300 lbs. of weight. To have this bar mounted, you need a door frame that sticks out of the wall. There has to be a ledge large enough to support the bar.

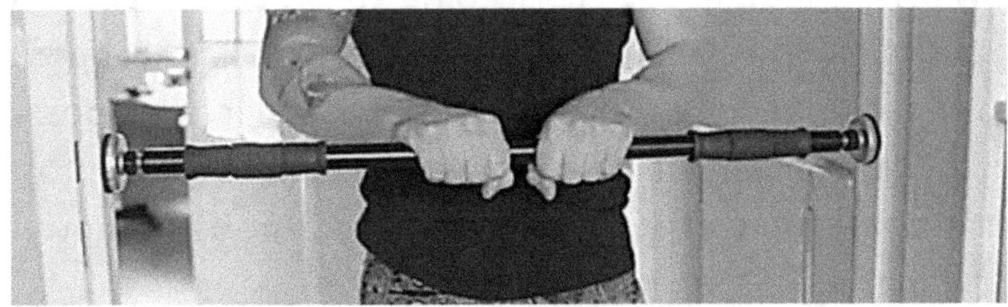

The above pull-up bar is the simplest and cheapest. It has screws in both ends, which can expand as you rotate it. It is very easy to set up, but has a couple of issues. You have to have a door frame that makes it possible to install the bar; certain door frames might be too thin for this equipment, and the bar would be good enough. Another thing to take into consideration is how sturdy the door frame and the wall are. If you want the bar to hold really well, you need to screw it in really strongly. This creates massive forces that can easily crack thinner walls or damage the door frame. On the other hand, if the bar isn't screwed in properly, it won't hold your weight, and you are risking damage.

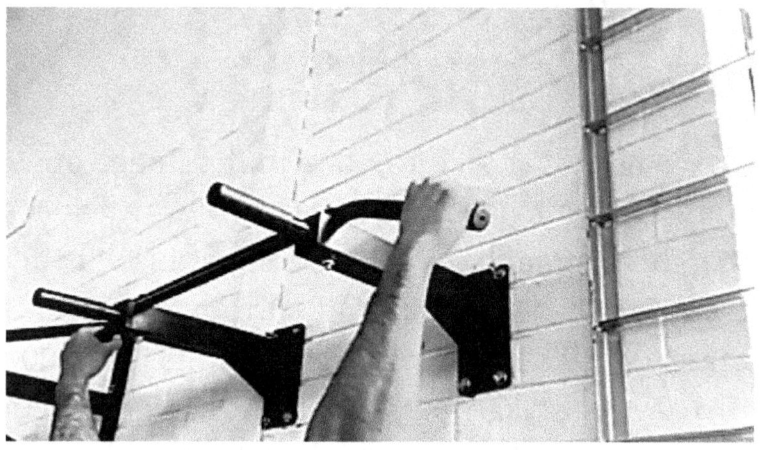

The bar above is one that can also be used if you can drill into the walls of your house; it is going to be stable and often inexpensive. However, it has its own flaws. These bars are usually positioned quite close to the wall, and it is not possible to train things like the front lever or back lever due to the limited space they offer. These bars can also be mounted to the ceiling.

Dips Bars

Dips stand out as one of the most effective exercises for specifically targeting your triceps. Within the realm of calisthenics, dips are considered indispensable due to their ability to engage not only the triceps but also the chest and core muscles, making them a highly efficient compound movement. The beauty of dip bars lies in their versatility; they can be conveniently utilized in various settings, including your home or workplace. While they do occupy some space, the benefits derived from this versatile piece of equipment are well worth it. Additionally, dip bars facilitate other fantastic exercises like Australian pull-ups and incline push-ups, further enhancing their utility in a comprehensive workout regimen.

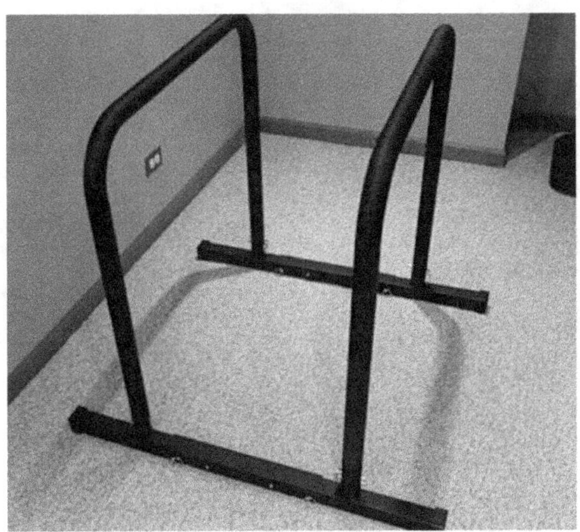

Parallettes

A close relative of the Dip Bar is the Parallette, which consists of two shorter parallel bars of smaller dimensions.

Calisthenics enthusiasts often employ Parallettes for honing their skills, including basic L-sits and handstand variations, as well as more challenging forms of push-ups. Furthermore, regular use of Parallettes can significantly enhance forearm and grip strength.

It's important to note that wooden Parallettes are favored for their comfort and skin-friendliness. Frequent use of plastic Parallettes, on the other hand, may eventually result in skin issues such as cuts and bruises. Therefore, opting for wooden Parallettes is a wise choice to ensure a more comfortable and injury-free training experience.

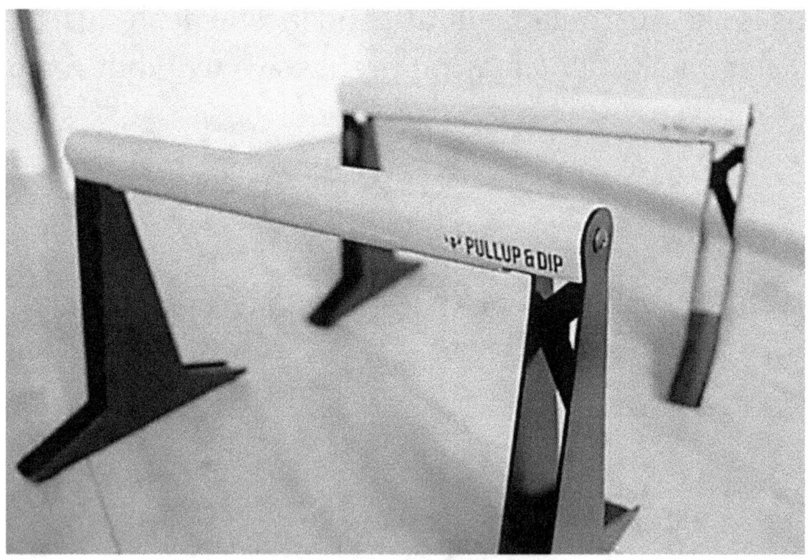

If you're seeking Parallettes that offer additional functionality, consider opting for taller ones, like the ones depicted in the image above. These taller Parallettes enable you to perform the same exercises as their smaller counterparts while providing extra features. They facilitate full-range handstand movements, allowing for more comprehensive training. Moreover, when positioned on top of a couple of chairs, these taller Parallettes even allow you to execute dips, expanding the range of exercises you can incorporate into your routine.

Resistance Bands

Resistance bands are invaluable tools that enable you to conquer challenging exercises that would typically be unattainable. These exercises include the renowned muscle-up, which demands exceptional upper- body strength and coordination. Both novice and seasoned calisthenics practitioners often employ resistance bands as a training aid when learning the muscle-up. They do so by looping the bands around the bar and their feet, which provides the assistance needed to master this demanding movement.

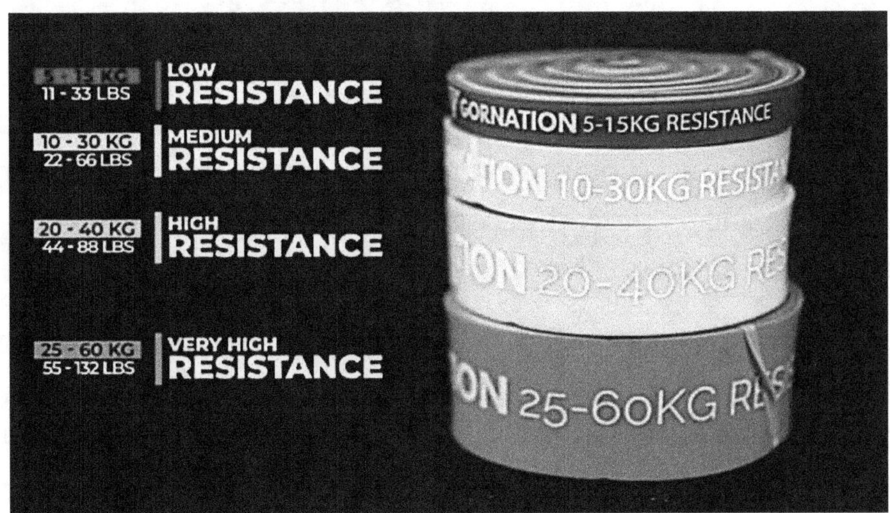

In this manner, the bands assist in partially offsetting the user's own body weight and facilitate the exercise. Your body will become accustomed to the action after a few repetitions of the workout with the bands, and you'll ultimately be able to complete it without them.

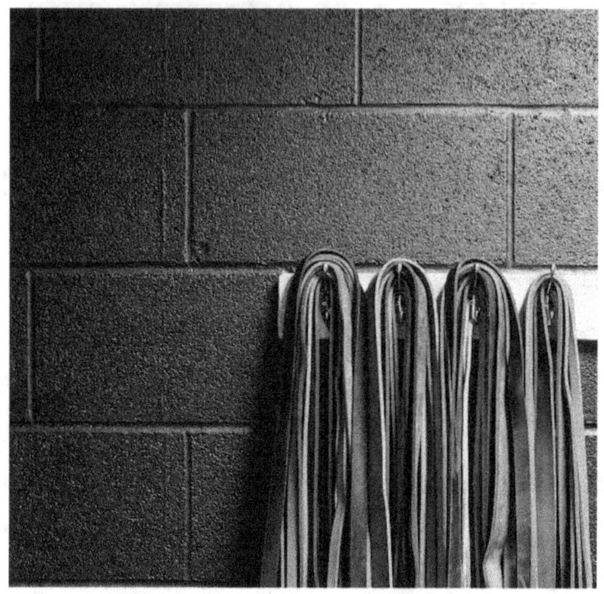

Traditional exercises such as push-ups and squats can be effectively intensified by incorporating resistance bands into your routine. By strategically placing the band around your back or shoulders, you can markedly increase the challenge of both the concentric and eccentric phases of these exercises, leading to enhanced strength gains.

Furthermore, resistance bands serve as valuable tools for warming up before your workout. Their versatility knows no bounds, with the potential for various applications limited only by your imagination and creativity. The options for incorporating resistance bands into your fitness regimen are virtually limitless.

Gymnastic Rings

Ever ponder why Olympic gymnasts are so powerful and muscular? Rings are the solution. They escalate the difficulty of each and every exercise. Try pushups, pullups, and dips using rings; you probably won't be able to do as many reps and sets as you usually can. When performing any workout, rings cause instability and make you feel unsteady.

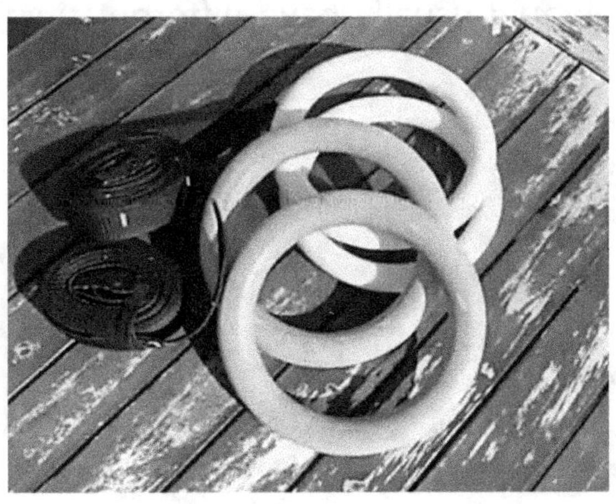

Again, wooden rings are recommended over plastic rings. Your skin will love you for it. Plastic rubs your skin in an unnecessary way, which may eventually result in more bruises and wounds.

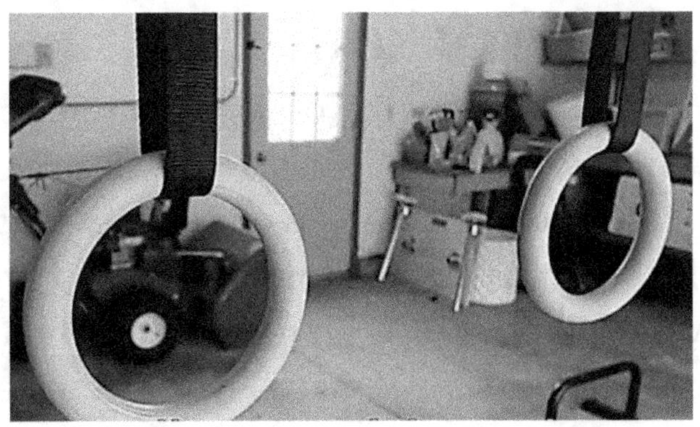

Massage Gun

A good massage gun will greatly reduce your recovery time and enable you to give your all throughout every training session. Use it at the very end of a workout or if you experience muscle soreness the day after a strenuous workout. As soon as you start experiencing the advantages, you'll develop an addiction to using your massager. The massage gun would usually have different tips for different muscle parts.

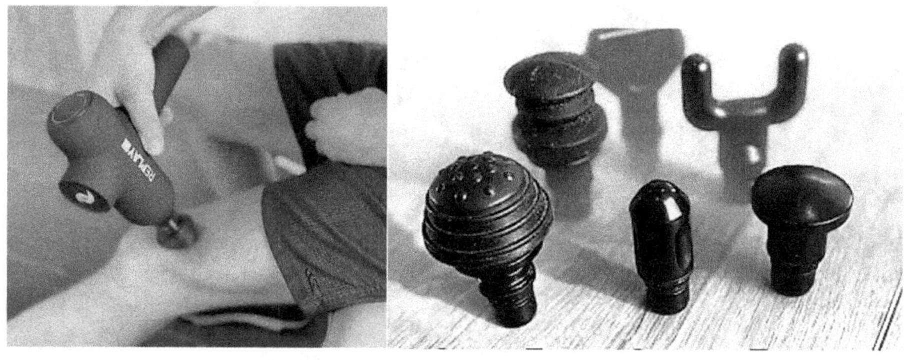

Make sure to experiment with the power and speed settings to find the one that makes you feel the most at ease. No single setting is ideal for everyone.

Workout Mat

Not only are these mats useful for yoga, but they can also be used for crunches, sit-ups, Russian twists, planks, mountain climbers, and a variety of other abs and core exercises. Unless you're at the beach or a park, doing things on hard surfaces will be very uncomfortable. Even then, using a mat will make you feel more at ease. A lot of mats have been tested, and the foldable exercise mat in the picture has been deemed the best. This mat is thick enough for comfort throughout all types of workouts, unlike many others that are too thin, and it's simple to put away after you're finished.

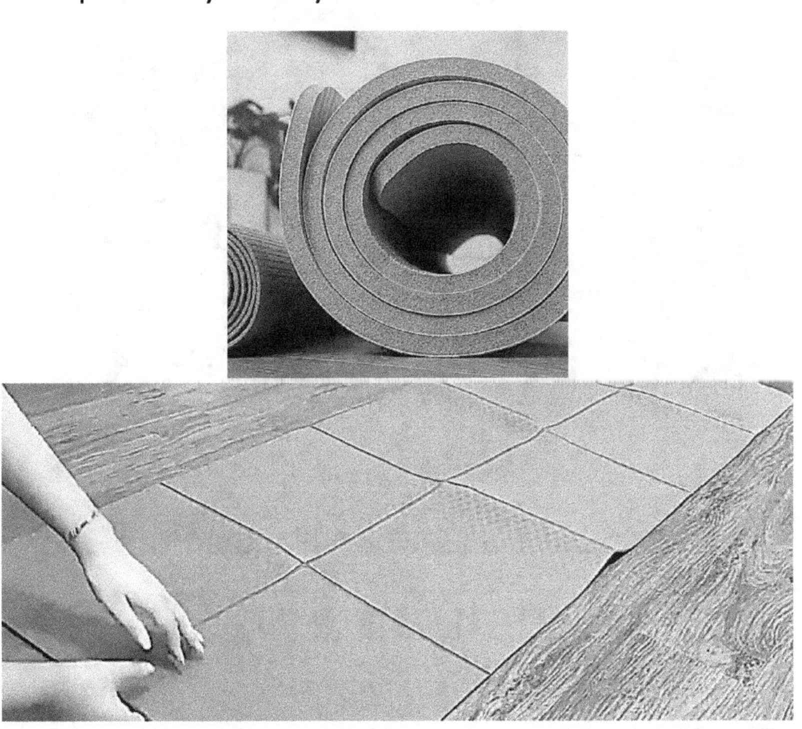

Chalk

Using liquid chalk while performing various workouts is a common way to strengthen your grip. Consider performing pull-ups as an example. Being able to complete the exercise depends heavily on having a firm grasp on the bar. Chalk can be helpful in this situation since it reduces the likelihood that your hands will be slick. Generally speaking, you should only apply the chalk to places that will be in contact with the bar. The goal is to delicately drag a block of chalk across your palm and along your fingers. It's not necessary to completely enclose your palms or shatter the chalk block in order to utilize it, for example. It would be a good idea to make plans to get some chalk if you plan to grip and hold objects a lot.

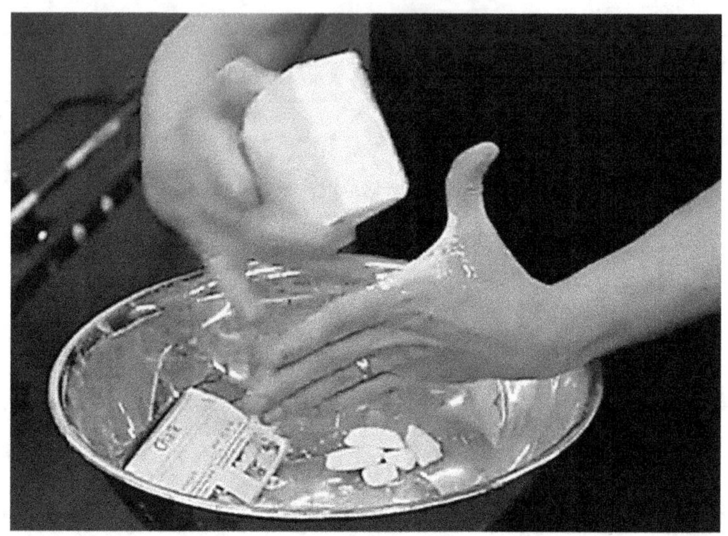

Push-up Bars

Push-up bars give another training benefit by extending the range of motion. They let you perform push-ups with a deeper downward action, which specifically stretches and strengthens the chest muscles even more. Push-ups are an extremely efficient exercise that also works the triceps, abdomen, shoulders, and buttocks in addition to the chest. Obviously, the handles are also the best handstand bar for practicing handstands in addition to push-ups.

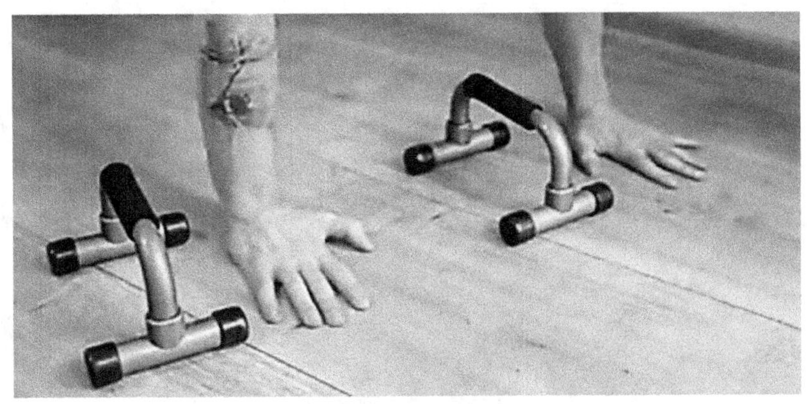

Gloves

When performing calisthenics, gloves can be quite useful because they will enable you to complete a variety of exercises. Calisthenics can be tough on your wrists and hands. Wearing the right gloves or pads can therefore be beneficial for reducing the chance of injuries and enhancing your overall grip.

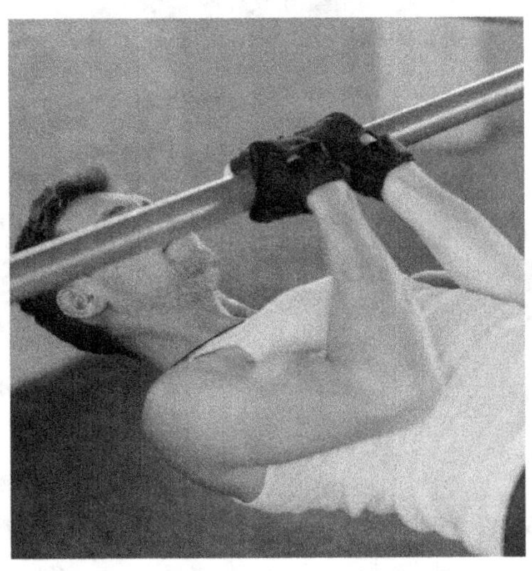

Jumping Rope

One of the best calisthenics tools you can purchase when starting out is a jumping rope. A lot of people have probably used one before, but if you haven't, you might still benefit from some simple tips.

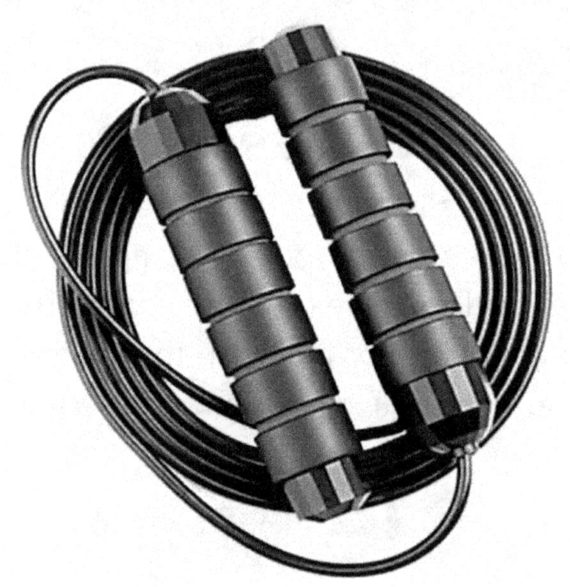

To begin, choose appropriate footwear when utilizing jumping ropes. Anything that makes it easier for you to move around should be considered. Second, practice in a space that is safe for movement and is sufficiently large to prevent congestion. This is to prevent accidentally hurting yourself or breaking objects.

In summary, it's of paramount importance to prioritize safety and proper usage when working with any fitness equipment. Take into account factors such as your hand grip, the quality of the equipment, the workout space, and the correct techniques for using the equipment.

Ultimately, calisthenics equipment can be a valuable and enriching component of your fitness routine, particularly for those embarking on their calisthenics journey. It's advisable to incorporate calisthenics equipment into your training regimen when starting out to reap its numerous benefits and build a strong foundation in this discipline.

About the Author

Bruce Nolan is a dedicated fitness enthusiast and a passionate advocate for calisthenics as a transformative fitness approach. With a background in exercise science and personal training, Bruce's journey into the world of calisthenics began as an exploration of functional movement and the incredible potential of bodyweight exercises.

Bruce's fitness philosophy centers around making exercise accessible to everyone, regardless of their fitness level or experience. His own journey from a novice to a calisthenics practitioner has given him valuable insights into the challenges beginners face. This empathetic understanding is at the heart of his writing and teaching.

As a certified personal trainer, Bruce possesses a deep understanding of exercise physiology and biomechanics. He blends this knowledge with a passion for helping individuals unleash their physical potential. Bruce's ability to break down complex movements into simple, actionable steps makes his writing ideal for those new to calisthenics.

With his book "Pure Calisthenics for Beginners," Bruce Nolan invites you to embark on a fitness journey that goes beyond the superficial. His relatable and informative writing style, combined with his real-world experience, makes him a trusted guide for beginners seeking to explore the world of calisthenics. Through Bruce's guidance, you'll not only learn the fundamentals of bodyweight exercises but also discover the power to rewrite your fitness story.